The Elephant in the Room

The Elephant in the Room

THE ULTIMATE GUIDE TO WEIGHT LOSS AND HEALTHY LIVING

Maha Abboud, MD and Terri Washington, MD

ISBN-13: 9781535240024
ISBN-10: 1535240024

Disclaimer

The opinions presented in this book are those of the authors. The authors make no guarantee regarding the contents of this book. The information described here is general and may not apply to a specific patient or person. Any product mentioned in this book should be taken according to the prescribing information provided by the manufacturer and in accordance with the advice of a prescribing physician.

Dedication

To all the people who have struggled with weight, past and present.

—TERRI WASHINGTON

Dedication

To the most amazing wonderful person in my life, my daughter Sabrina.

To the bright stars in my life- my nephews, Michael, Kais, Maher, Firas, Johnnie; and my nieces, Bana, Petra and Aria.

To my parents—for their never-ending love and support

To my husband, Steve, whose support helped bring the words from my head to the paper

To my sister Mahassen, who like the bamboo tree, blooms wherever she is planted

To the angels of the earth—my sisters Elham and Nazek

To the one who never stops fighting—my sister Rinati

To the cornerstones of my life—my brothers, Ghassan and Amer

To the one who stood by me through thick and thin—my brother-in-law Maan

To the ones who never lost hope—my fellow Syrians

—MAHA ABBOUD

Contents

CHAPTER 1
Introduction: The State of Things

As endocrinologists or hormone doctors, we see hundreds of people each week, and the biggest complaint we hear is "I want to lose weight" or "Doc, I just can't seem to lose weight, no matter what I do." Often, with a combination of medications, changes in lifestyle and diet, and correction of underlying hormonal abnormalities, our patients can lose weight. However, there are a lot of misconceptions about obesity. People do not really understand the cause or what it really takes to lose weight and keep it off. Each year millions of people make resolutions to eat healthier and exercise more. However, they do not take into consideration the many factors working against them. "It just takes some willpower" or "Why don't you just eat less" are some of the things we tell ourselves. Sadder still is the fact that the advice that many people get from their doctors, if they get advice at all, is to "Cut back" or "Stop eating so much." People hear this also from their loved ones who do not understand the support that is needed or the changes that are necessary to really lose weight. We want you to understand that overeating is not the only reason for weight gain.

For these reasons we wrote this book to help people understand exactly what being overweight and being obese mean. Although energy imbalance contributes to weight gain, we want you to know that it is not only lifestyle, lack of exercise, and diet that are contributing to the obesity epidemic in this country. Obesity is a complex chronic disease. Note the word *disease*. That means there are defects in the body system that cause changes in hormones and metabolism that affect weight. This determines how easy (or difficult) it is to lose weight or maintain a certain weight. In this book we will explore what obesity means, what causes obesity, and what steps can be taken to combat it.

CHAPTER 2

Obesity: What Is It, and What's the Cause?

The public has long held the belief that obesity was something that a person causes or does to him- or herself. If you did not eat so much, you would not be fat. If you exercised more, you could keep the weight off. First it is important to understand exactly what obesity is. Obesity, simply put, means having too much fat. As physicians we characterize obesity based on the body mass index (BMI). BMI is a ratio of one's weight compared to height. It is an easy measure to calculate and has been in use as the standard for identifying obesity by the World Health Organization (WHO) since the 1980s. A normal BMI ranges from eighteen to twenty-four. A person is considered overweight if his or her BMI is twenty-five to twenty-nine, and a BMI greater than thirty is considered obese. Although this number is not perfect, we use it because it helps us to determine a person's risk for various diseases and health problems such as prediabetes, diabetes, joint pain, and heart disease, among other problems. BMI does not take into account, however, factors such as muscularity and is inaccurate for the very athletic and muscular. Despite this, it is useful for most people. Figure 2 shows the classification of obesity and risk level associated with each waist circumference (WC) and BMI.

Another measure that better identifies the risk of disease from obesity is WC. WC identifies visceral fat. This is the fat in the middle that surrounds organs and causes problems when in excess. Visceral fat is different from subcutaneous (SC) fat. SC fat is fat that sits under the skin. Excessive visceral fat is considered central obesity. SC fat is also "metabolically active." It produces and releases hormones that affect blood sugar, inflammation, and how cholesterol is metabolized and stored. When there is an overabundance of fat, it gets deposited around the internal organs such as the liver, spleen, kidneys, and pancreas. It releases substances that cause inflammation and can lead to liver disease, prediabetes or worsening diabetes, and plaque formation in the arteries.

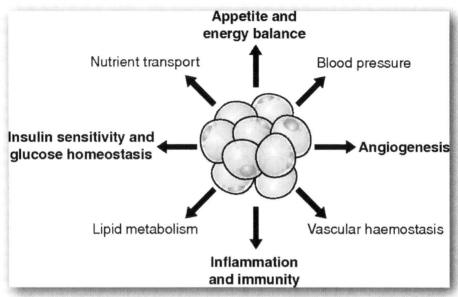

Figure 1. Illustration of the various metabolic and hormone pathways that adipose (fat) tissue controls.

Image retrieved from: *Physiological Reviews* 93 (1): 1–21. doi:10.1152/physrev.00017.2012. Published January 1, 2013.

This image demonstrates that fat tissue produces and secretes hormones and other substance that control not only diet, energy storage, and nutrient transport but also blood pressure, cholesterol or lipid metabolism, inflammation, insulin and blood sugar control, and angiogenesis, which is the development of new blood vessels necessary to carry nutrients to various tissues.

According to the National Heart, Lung, and Blood Institute (NHLBI), a division of the National Institute of Health (NIH), WC and BMI are related, but WC "provides independent risk over and above that of BMI." This is especially useful for identifying people at risk for disease who have normal weight or are overweight according to BMI measurement. As noted in the NHLBI obesity guidelines textbook, a high waist circumference is associated with an increased risk of type 2 diabetes, high cholesterol, hypertension, and heart disease in patients with a BMI between 25 and 34.9. Waist circumference is measured at the top of the iliac crest, with the tape measure held snug, at the end of normal expiration (see figure 3). People with a waist circumference measurement above normal should be considered at higher risk than their BMI would suggest.

Body-fat percentage is also a useful measure of adiposity or obesity. It is the total body-fat mass divided by the total weight. Body fat consists of necessary (essential) body fat, needed to sustain life and reproductive functions, and storage fat, which is needed for energy storage. Men have essential body fat of 2–5 percent; and women, 10–13 percent (Apovian, Arrone, and Powell 2015). Normal total body-fat percentages vary depending on sex, ethnicity, and age, but in general, the normal range for men is 10–24 percent; and for women, 21–27 percent. There are a number of ways to measure body fat and, consequently, health risk. These include skinfold analysis with calipers, bioelectrical impedance analysis, and dual-energy x-ray absorption (DEXA). These methods are done either by trainers at the gym or can be found in some doctors' offices and, in the case of DEXA, are used in research. See chapter 10 for further information on body composition and measurement of fat percentage.

Table 1. Classification of overweight and obesity by body mass index (BMI), waist circumference, and associated disease risk.

	BMI (kg/m^2)	Obesity class	Disease risk[a] relative to normal weight and waist circumference	
			Men ≤ 102 cm (≤ 40 in.) Women ≤ 88 cm (≤ 35 in.)	> 102 cm (> 40 in.) > 88 cm (> 35 in.)
Underwieight	< 18.5		-	-
Normal[b]	18.5 - 24.9		-	-
Overweight	25.0 - 29.9		Increased	High
Obesity	30.0 - 34.9	I	High	Very high
	35.0 - 39.9	II	Very high	Very high
Extreme obesity	≥ 40	III	Extremely high	Extremely high

a) Disease risk for type 2 diabetes mellitus, hypertension, and cardiovascular disease.

b) Increased waist circumference also can be a marker for increased risk even in persons of normal weight.

From World Health Organ Technical Report Series 894 (2000): i–xii, 1–253 [7].

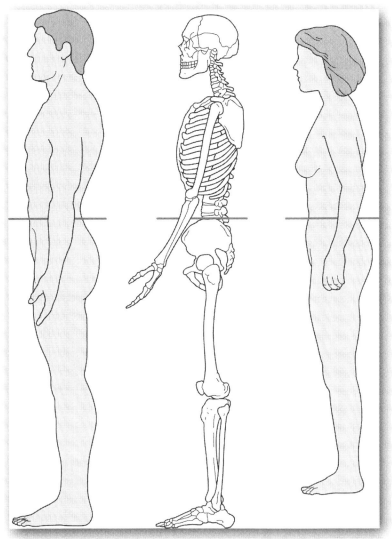

Figure 2. Measuring tape position for waist (abdominal) circumference.

High Risk
Men: >102 cm (>40 in.)
Women: >88 cm (>35 in.)

http://www.nhlbi.nih.gov/health-pro/guidelines/current/obesity-guidelines/e_textbook/txgd/4142.htm#content

Obesity is a chronic disease. A disease is a disorder of structure or function that can produce specific signs or symptoms. In 2013, the American Medical Association, the American Association of Clinical Endocrinologists, and the Endocrine Society worked to get obesity recognized as a disease. The American Heart Association, American College of Cardiology, and The Obesity Society released guidelines in November 2013 stating doctors should treat obesity as a disease and actively treat obese patients with weight-loss recommendations and medications as indicated. According to Gordon Tomaselli, MD, a former president of the American heart association, "The subsequent health problems of obesity and the risk factors in a person's family history passed down through the generations have become increasingly more of a burden. That's the siren sound we can no longer ignore." Why is this important? If doctors do not recognize the problem, then we are less likely to discuss it with patients and offer them possible treatments. Doctors may not have interest in treating obesity because in the past, few options were available. Also several medicines used for weight-loss treatment in the past caused serious side effects such as heart disease and were taken off the market. If insurance companies do not recognize obesity as a disease, they do not have to pay for treatment. They can deny medications and life-saving surgical treatment to those who need it most. More insurance companies are starting to offer coverage for obesity treatment, but coverage is still varied and not widespread. The good news is that new medication treatments are available, and for select people, surgery is a good treatment option. The practical approach to obesity is one that addresses the patient's concerns and includes combination therapy with diet, exercise, medications, and surgery if recommended. We have come a long way in regards to surgical options for weight loss (see chapter 12).

In the United States alone, 78.6 million adults are obese. That is greater than one-third of the population (34.9 percent) according to the Center for Disease Control (CDC) website (Ogden et al. 2014). The percentage of obese Americans has tripled since 1960 to its current prevalence today. The number of obese children and morbidly (severe) obese adults has increased as well (Flegal et al. 2002).

Obesity prevalence in 2014 varies across states and territories. Consider the following:

- No state had a prevalence of obesity less than 20 percent.
- Five states and the District of Columbia had a prevalence of obesity between 20 and 25 percent.
- Twenty-three states, Guam, and Puerto Rico had a prevalence of obesity between 25 and 30 percent.

- Nineteen states had a prevalence of obesity between 30 and 35 percent.
- Three states (Arkansas, Mississippi, and West Virginia) had a prevalence of obesity of 35 percent or greater.
- The Midwest had the highest prevalence of obesity (30.7 percent), followed by the South (30.6 percent), the Northeast (27.3 percent), and the West (25.7 percent).

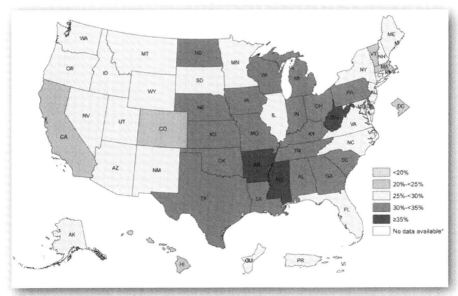

Figure 3. Prevalence of Self-Reported Obesity among US
Adults by State and Territory, BRFSS, 2014.

Prevalence estimates reflect BRFSS methodological changes started in 2011.
These estimates should not be compared to prevalence estimates before 2011.

Source: Behavioral Risk Factor Surveillance System, CDC. http://www.cdc.gov/
obesity/data/prevalence-maps.html.

These numbers are worse for minorities. Non-Hispanic blacks have the highest rates of obesity (47.8 percent), followed by Hispanics (42.5 percent), non-Hispanic whites (32.6 percent), and Asians (10.8 percent). Middle-aged adults forty to fifty-nine years old have higher rates of obesity (39.5 percent) compared to younger adults, aged twenty to thirty-nine (30.3 percent), or adults over the age of sixty (35.4 percent) (Ogden et al. 2014). No matter what your ethnicity is, you are not alone in the struggle. The sadder fact is that obesity affects children as well. The *Journal of the American Medical Association* reported in 2014 that from the years 2011 to 2012, 17 percent (12.7 million) of children between the ages of two and nineteen were obese (CDC 2015). The cost of America's expanding waistline affects not only our wallets at the clothing store but also our health and life-span. The risks of being overweight and obese include, but are not limited to, developing diabetes, heart disease, cancer, gallbladder disease, osteoarthritis, gout, and sleep apnea. Overweight women may have menstrual problems and infertility. Obese men are more likely to have low testosterone with resulting fatigue, muscle weakness, and loss of libido. Obese children grow up to become obese adults with the same problems and can develop diabetes earlier in life.

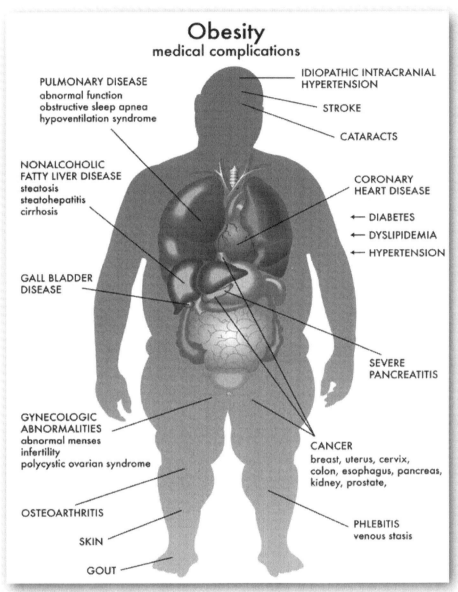

Figure 4. Diagram of medical complications of obesity. Image retrieved from http://www.healthinfocus.net/blog/obesita/.

What causes obesity? There are a number of factors that contribute to a person's weight. Age, diet, activity, genetics, medications, and hormones determine what weight you maintain. There are factors that we can control, like what we eat and how much we exercise, but there are also factors that we cannot control, such as cultural influences, socioeconomic status, and our genes. Things around us that influence our weight, such as easily available, high-calorie, highly enjoyable foods that stimulate the brain's reward centers, lead to food intake even without hunger. Think about how many times you have been out to eat and became full but kept eating because the food was so good. Have you ever been at a party and could not resist a piece of cake or a plate because of the pressure of family and friends asking why you were not eating? Some encourage you to eat, saying, "It's OK; it's for a special occasion" or "Go ahead; it's just this one piece." On top of the pressure to eat and the irresistible desire for tasty foods, many jobs today are sedentary and require low levels of activity, so people burn fewer calories throughout the day. Stress and lack of sleep often make you want to eat more. Our jobs, particularly those with shift changes, affect the natural body clock and contribute to hunger and weight gain. Also, as people age, their metabolism slows each decade. That means you expend less energy as you age despite the same level of activity or intake of calories, which makes it difficult to lose weight with age. One has to eat less and exercise more just to maintain a certain weight as they age. Other factors such as medications can play a part. Several medications have weight gain as a side effect.

Medicines vary in the amount and ability to cause weight gain, and often the mechanism of weight gain is not clearly understood. Nonetheless if you need a medication for treatment, you should take it as directed. However, you should be aware of the possible side effects of the medication. If weight gain is a concern, talk to your doctor to see if an alternative is available. When no alternative is available, the minimal dose needed to produce the desired effect should be taken. Drug-induced weight gain can be preventable. When possible, choose medications that are weight neutral or cause weight loss (Apovian, Arrone, and Powell 2015). As physicians we try to balance the desired clinical effect with side effects that include weight gain in particular with diabetic patients, as weight gain worsens diabetes. As a patient it is your job to be informed of potential side effects and to become educated on weight management (from portion control to regular exercise). Here we discuss a few common medications known to lead to weight gain, and below is a chart of these meds and list of alternatives.

Table 2. Examples of commonly used drugs that cause weight gain, are weight neutral, or cause weight loss.

Weight Gain	Weight Neutral	Weight Loss
Antidepressants		
Nortriptyline Doxepin Amitriptyline, Imipramine Phenelzine Paroxetine Citalopram Fluoxetine (greater than one year)	Bupropion Fluoxetine(less than one year) Sertraline (less than one year) Nefazodone	Bupropion
Sertraline (greater than one year) Mirtazapine		
Antihypertensives		
Prazosin Doxazosin Metoprolol tartrate Propranolol Atenolol	Carvedilol Nebivolol	

Weight Gain	Weight Neutral	Weight Loss
Antidiabetics		

Insulin
Sulfonylureas
Thiazolidinediones
(rosiglitazone and
pioglitazone)
	Alpha-glucosidase
	inhibitors
	Acarbose
	(Precose)
	Miglitol (glycet)
	DPP-4 inhibitors
	(sitagliptin, vida-
	gliptin, saxagliptin,
	alogliptin)
		Metformin
		GLP-1 agonists
		    (Exenatide, lira-
		glutide, dulaglutide)
		Pramlinitde
		Sodium glucose
		cotransporter 2
		(SGLT-2) inhibitors
		    (canagliflozin,
		dapagliflozin,
		emapgliflozin)

Antiepileptics		
Gabapentin Pregabalin Valproic acid Vigabatrin Carbamazepine	Lamotrigine Levetiracetam Phenytoin	Felbamate Topiramate Zonisamide
Contraceptives and Hormones		
Depo- medroxyprogesterone acetate (Depo-Provera) Megestrol acetate (not contraceptive but is a hormone used for weight gain)		

Anithistamines		
Diphenhydramine Meclizine Cyproheptadine		
Antipsychotics		
Clozapine Olanzapine Risperidone Quetiapine Perphenazine Lithium	Ziprasidone Aripiprazole	
Steroids		
Glucocorticoids Progestins		

When it comes to diabetes, insulin, sulfonylureas, and thiazolidine-diones (TZDs) are the most common medicines that cause weight gain. The amount of weight gain is dose dependent, particularly with insulin. Insulin appears to cause more weight gain than oral medications. Weight gain due to sulfonylureas is due to increase in insulin secretion and is approximately two pounds per year. TZDs cause weight gain by different mechanisms and can lead to fluid retention. There are other medications available for diabetes that are weight neutral or can cause weight loss. These should be considered first when possible.

Other common medicines known to cause weight gain are steroids and oral contraceptives, which are estrogen and progesterone hormones. Steroids are used for a number of acute and chronic inflammatory illnesses, such as asthma, arthritis, and vasculitis. The higher the dose and the longer the medications are used, even intermittently, the more weight gained. Nonsteroidal anti-inflammatory drugs should be used when possible. Women often are concerned that they will gain weight when starting birth control and hormone therapy, and this can influence whether women take the medication and stay on it. The weight gain seen with birth-control pills is variable, from one to seventeen pounds over one year. The studies on birth-control pills and weight gain have shown inconsistent results. Some studies show significant weight gain with oral contraceptives while other studies fail to show definite increases in weight after several cycles (Rosenberg 1998; Vrbikova et al. 2006). Hormonal changes also contribute to the defects that cause weight gain. As endocrinologists, we see a lot of diabetic patients, and over the years we have learned of the core defects of diabetes referred to as the ominous octet. This refers to eight major defects in different organ systems that contribute to high blood sugar and ultimately diabetes. Similarly one can think of an obesity octet for obesity/weight gain. This includes the following:

1. **Insulin resistance**

2. **Amylin resistance**

3. **Ghrelin**

4. **Glucagon-like peptide (GLP-1) resistance**

5. **Peptide YY (PYY) resistance**

6. **Leptin resistance**

7. **Serotonin activity**

8. **Dopamine abnormality**

The image below shows that adipose tissue and hormones secreted from the gut signal the brain to regulate feeding and hunger. There are a number of areas for potential hormone imbalances that can affect the appetite and thus food intake.

Each of these hormones plays a role in how hungry or full you feel. They affect your ability to keep weight off and affect food intake differently before and after weight loss. This is why people are often able to lose weight but tend to regain weight soon after weight loss. The human body has evolved to maintain a steady state of balance, or energy homeostasis. This is a balance between energy taken in by food and drink and energy used, or burned, with activity and bodily functions. Your body wants to maintain its weight and does so through complex communication between the brain and the organs like the gut (Apovian, Arrone, and Powell 2015). In order to maintain balance, the brain senses fuel availability (nutrients) and produces signals to control food intake and energy expenditure. Under normal balanced conditions, all the fuel or energy consumed is used to maintain the basal metabolic rate, heat production, and energy use. Any excess fuel is stored as fat to be used later as needed, particularly in times of starvation.

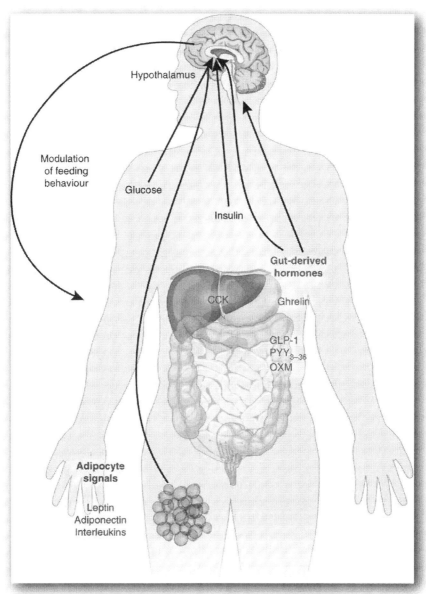

Figure 5. Hormones secreted in the gut and adipose
tissue affect the brain and feeding behavior.

Image retrieved from http://www.nature.com/neuro/
journal/v15/n10/fig_tab/nn.3211_F2.html.

CHAPTER 3

My Hormones Do *What?*

What is a hormone? It is a substance produced by the body that is transported through the bloodstream to tissues where it has a specific effect. There are numerous hormones that control various bodily functions in the same way traffic lights work. Think about driving without traffic lights and how difficult commuting to and from work would be without them. Some drivers would move too slow and frustrate you, and others would drive too fast. Either way there are likely to be many accidents or traffic jams. That is how the body would function without balanced hormones. Hormones facilitate communication among different organs and help to control different functions of the body. Hormonal function is a complicated thing. It can be difficult to tease out the exact hormonal problem, but it is not impossible. Patients who suffer from obesity may have low or excess hormone levels. There can be resistance to hormones in the body, and sometimes hormones are needed to treat different problems.

A common hormone people like to blame for weight gain is the thyroid hormone. While the thyroid affects metabolism and metabolic rate, it is not a common cause of weight gain. Changes in hormones secreted from fat tissue, the stomach, the gut, and the pancreas signal the brain to regulate food intake and the amount of energy the body burns. All these hormones work together in a complex fashion, and problems can occur on various levels and act in a way that leads to weight gain.

The pancreas produces insulin and amylin. Typically when one thinks of insulin, one thinks of blood-sugar control. Insulin has other functions and helps to promote the storage of energy as fat. Fasting-insulin levels correlate with fat mass, meaning that the higher the insulin levels, the more fat one is likely to have. When levels are altered, it leads to increased hunger. Amylin similar to a hormone *leptin* binds to neurons in the brain leading to decreased food intake (Apovian, Arrone, and Powell 2015). Amylin is a hormone that is secreted with insulin and, along with insulin, helps to lower blood sugar. In addition, it slows digestion and the emptying of the stomach after a meal. It also helps to increase satiety or feelings of fullness. This not only helps to decrease glucose (blood sugar) spikes after meals but also contributes to satiety and eating less. Obese patients often have either decreased levels or resistance to various hormones, which leads to increased hunger and food intake.

Ghrelin is the hunger hormone. It is produced in the stomach and acts quickly on the brain to initiate food intake. Ghrelin levels are elevated during times of fasting and fall quickly with eating. The problem comes when a person tries to cut back on calories or increase exercise. The body says, "Hey, what is going on?" and ghrelin levels increase, leading to increased hunger in order for the body to maintain its current weight. In contrast to ghrelin is leptin. Leptin is produced by fat cells and leads to decreased food intake and early satiety. It signals the brain that fat stores are sufficient. Leptin levels are low in starvation, but in obese patients, levels of leptin are increased, suggesting resistance to leptin. As a result, obese people do not have normal feelings of fullness despite higher levels of leptin.

The gut produces several hormones such as GLP-1, CCK, PYY, and serotonin, which act in various ways to decrease intake and signal satiety. CCK is released in the duodenum and small intestines in response to fat and protein intake. GLP-1 and PYY are released from the small intestines in response to nutrient stimulation. GLP-1 slows the stomach from emptying quickly and leads to earlier feelings of fullness, whereas the other hormones signal to the brain, causing satiety. PYY levels rise with eating, and it signals food intake in the gut and satiety in the brain. Levels of PYY drop with weight loss, and this leads to less fullness and increased hunger, which in turn contributes to weight regain.

In developed countries today, there is an overabundance of food and options. Snack foods and meals that have high sugar and fat content are easy to obtain and often trigger the brain's reward center, leading to addictive behavior. According to Apovian, Arrone, and Powell (2015) obesity and the obesity epidemic may in part be driven by the "excessive motivational drive for food" and mediated by the reward "hedonic" pathway, which involves hormones and neurotransmitters like serotonin, dopamine, and catecholamine. The response to food is complex, due to a number of factors that contribute to food intake and food choices in people. Taste along with "availability, economics, incentives ('supersizing') and social routines" influence what and how much we eat, write Apovian, Arrone, and Powell (2015) During times of energy abundance, the brain's reward system can override the steady-state homeostatic mechanisms that control hunger and intake by increasing the desire to consume good-tasting, pleasing foods even when hunger is not present (Apovian, Arrone, and Powell 2015). For example, have you ever found yourself eating a cookie but could not stop at one? The next thing you know, you have eaten the whole bag and are not sure how it happened. You are not alone, and this is in part due to chemical reactions in the brain. Several neurotransmitters, substances that lead to communication between neurons, are involved in the rewarding or addictive attraction to food (Apovian, Arrone, and Powell 2015). Dopamine and serotonin are two examples of such neurotransmitters. Dopamine has been the most studied. Studies using magnetic resonance imaging (MRI) have shown increased activation in areas of the brain that release dopamine in response to highly palatable foods. The increased activity was greater for obese patients compared to normal-weight patients. This also was seen in response to pictures of high-calorie foods like cake and ribs versus low-calorie foods like vegetables and broiled fish (Stoeckel et al. 2008).

Excessive reactions to high-calorie foods might play an underlying role in obesity today. Obese people may have a hyperactive reward system making food more rewarding and leading to increased intake.

CHAPTER 4

Stress and Weight Gain

We all know that stress takes a toll on our daily lives, but many of us do not realize the significant impact that stress can have on our body. Specifically, we do not pay attention to the impact that stress has on our body's function, particularly when it comes to weight.

It is important to remember that external factors cause internal responses, and if you are dealing with excessive amounts of stress, realize that your body is working hard in response to that stress. When dealing with stress, our bodies make short-term adjustments in order to optimize their ability to respond to a variety of threats. However, one thing the body is not very good at is dealing with chronic stress over a long period of time. This is how many of us live our daily lives—under significant amounts of stress. Here we discuss a few ways that your body actively responds to stress and how that response could affect your weight.

Our mind and body are very good at quickly processing and reacting to significant threats. It is arguably one of the main reasons our species has survived and continues to thrive. Our ability to react and respond to stress has evolved and improved over time; however, our bodies are not good at maintaining reactions to stress over sustained periods of time.

We have all heard of the fight-or-flight response, when our mind and body quickly evaluate a threat and then make a decision whether to stay and fight or run and live to fight another day. While we typically think of this reaction as a response to physical threats, like being chased by a large animal or attacker, our bodies have a much more difficult time making that distinction. The body responds to mental threats, like dealing with difficult coworkers or actively stressing over a deadline at work, the same way it does to physical threats.

Whether dealing with a physical or mental stressor, the body's response is controlled by its ability to regulate hormones, like adrenaline, in order to improve awareness and specific bodily functions. While most responses are great in the short term, increased hormonal responses over long periods of time can have significant impacts and long-term effects on the body.

Our body responds to acute, short-term stress by increasing the production of the adrenaline hormone. This response has an immediate impact on the body, such as increasing heart rate and blood pressure, expanding air passages, increasing blood flow to the muscles, enlarging pupils, and much more. Basically the body is preparing for anything and everything, affecting every major system in your body.

Cortisol secretion increases in the body, along with adrenaline. Cortisol is a stress hormone that regulates energy in the body, including blood glucose. This is important because during increased periods of stress (short and long term), the body adjusts cortisol levels to ensure it has enough energy to survive the threat. Then the body naturally looks for ways to refill energy that has been lost due to increased adrenaline and cortisol, even if there has been little to no energy loss.

Imagine that your body is preparing to deal with a significant physical threat (e.g., running from a dog). Even if your stress is due to a work deadline, which requires significantly less energy output than running from a dog, your body would respond the same way and begin looking for ways to refill its energy or fuel reserves. This need to restock energy reserves results in increased food cravings, even if you are not really hungry or calorie deficient. Unfortunately, as we deal with continuous stress on a daily, weekly, and even monthly basis, our body continues to respond by storing energy as fat even though the needs and responses to most of our daily stressors are not physical.

In addition to increased fat storage, stress has other significant effects on the body and its many systems. Metabolism, digestion, blood glucose, cholesterol, fertility, and many more systems are affected. As you can see, understanding the body and how it works makes it much easier to identify the issues that could be causing weight gain and/or hindering your ability to lose weight. Working with a doctor can help you identify and address these issues that are impacting your short-term and long-term health.

Below is a figure of various strategies and treatments used for weight loss; medications and surgical options will be elaborated on in later chapters.

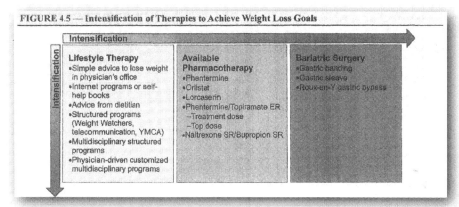

FIGURE 4.5 — Intensification of Therapies to Achieve Weight Loss Goals

Figure 6. This figure demonstrates the steps taken to lose weight, from less intense therapy to adding medications after lifestyle changes and finally surgery as the most intense therapy, after other methods have failed (Apovian, Arrone, and Powell 2015).

CHAPTER 5

What Does My Blood Sugar Have to Do with My Weight? Diabetes, Prediabetes, and Obesity

Being overweight or obese increases the risk of developing prediabetes and type 2 diabetes. Excess weight and high blood sugar are linked. If you recall, visceral fat is an endocrine organ. It secretes hormones and substances that affect the metabolism of sugar and fat and lead to inflammation. This is important to understand, because every 6.6 pounds of weight gain (or a one-unit increase in BMI) increases the risk of diabetes by approximately 12 percent. The majority of diabetes risk is attributed to excess weight. To put it another way, 68–72 percent of the risk of developing diabetes is from being overweight or obese (Ford, Williamson, and Liu 1997). According to the CDC, the number of people with type 2 diabetes has tripled in the last thirty years, in large part due to the obesity epidemic. The 2014 National Diabetes Statistics reported that twenty-nine million Americans have diabetes. Even more, eighty-six million adults have prediabetes, which is up from fifty-seven million in 2009 (http://www.cdc.gov/features/diabetesfactsheet/).

So what makes someone a prediabetic or puts him or her at risk for diabetes? One diagnostic factor is the hemoglobin A1C level. This is what doctors use to evaluate blood-sugar control. The A1C is a three-month average of the blood sugar. A hemoglobin A1C of ≤5.6 percent is normal. A person with an A1C of 5.7–6.4 percent is considered prediabetic, and one with an A1C greater than 6.5 percent is considered diabetic. Another thing we evaluate people for is metabolic syndrome. It is a cluster of abnormal values that identifies people at risk for developing diabetes and complications of obesity. Metabolic syndrome is recognized by the National Cholesterol Education Program (NCEP), CDC, and AACE. There are five criteria, and meeting three of the five gives one diagnosis of metabolic syndrome. The first criterion is abdominal obesity, or central fat, measured by WC. The cut-off is a WC >40 inches (102 cm) in men and >35 inches (88 cm) in women. Second is the triglyceride (type of fat) level: >150; third is the HDL (good cholesterol): <40 in men and <50 in women. Fourth is blood pressure: >130/85, and fifth is a fasting blood sugar >100.

All of these risk factors are related to obesity and future health complications. Patients with metabolic syndrome have a cycle of disease onset, worsening risk, and progression to diabetes and heart disease. We see people at various stages in our practice. Teenagers may present with excessive acne and weight gain. Females may present with irregular periods and develop polycystic ovarian syndrome, which includes insulin resistance and metabolic syndrome as a component. As women get older, they can develop infertility due to excess weight and hormone abnormalities, and if they do become pregnant, they are at risk for gestational diabetes and birth defects if the blood sugar is high during pregnancy. During middle-aged years, women and men present with obesity, high blood pressure, and are more likely to have diabetes. In the sixth and seventh decade, they present with heart disease and stroke. Because of the serious potential health risk, it is our responsibility as physicians to identify patients at various times in their life who are at risk and who meet the criteria for metabolic syndrome, prediabetes or who present with signs of hormonal abnormalities that may be related to insulin resistance. This is our opportunity to educate patients and discuss with them changes they can make early on, if possible, to decrease risk of diabetes, heart disease, and stroke. It is the time to discuss with people their weight, risk factors, and the things that can be done to change these things before it is too late.

The good news is that weight loss has been shown to control blood sugar, hypertension, and decrease the risk of heart disease associated with not only diabetes but also metabolic syndrome. Why is this? The more visceral fat tissue one has, the more it releases adipokines and hormones that signal inflammation and decrease insulin sensitivity. Loss of this fat mass leads to improvement in sugar metabolism and insulin sensitivity. In other words, tissues use insulin better, and blood-sugar control is improved. It does not require large amounts of weight loss. Small to moderate amounts of weight loss make a big improvement in health. In our practice, we have witnessed people who have been able to decrease or stop insulin and stop even oral diabetic medicine with changes in the diet and weight loss. Improvement in diabetes and prediabetes occurs early with weight loss. It has been shown that a decrease in body weight by only 5–7 percent improves not only the blood-sugar control but also the control of high blood pressure (Khaodhiar, Cummings, and Apovian 2009).

CHAPTER 6
An Individual Approach to Weight Loss

Have you ever asked why your friend or relative can lose weight and you cannot? The answer is: no two people are the same, and often people hit roadblocks and give up on weight loss. Factors that affect patients and doctors alike when dealing with and discussing weight loss include time limitations; feeling of discomfort talking about weight; and the lack of knowledge on nutrition, activity, and medication options. As mentioned before, there are a number of factors that contribute to weight, the ability to lose weight, and weight regain. For example, genes that contribute to obesity have been identified. People who have two copies of the FTO gene weigh on average six to nine pounds more than those without the gene. Those with one copy have reported increased food intake and decreased satiety (Timpson et al. 2008). Physical, social, economic, and environmental factors all contribute to obesity. Physical things such as easy access to transportation as well as exposure to pesticides and pollutants that cause hormonal changes contribute to weight gain. Social factors that influence meal duration, amount of food consumed, and advertisements for food and larger portions all affect the population's expanding waistline (Apovian, Arrone, and Powell 2015). Additionally many medical conditions as well as medications can cause weight gain.

According to data from the National Health and Nutrition Examination Survey, 2009–10, more than two out of three people in the United States are overweight; greater than one out of three are obese, and greater than one of twenty are extremely obese. In other words, more than two-thirds of the population is either overweight or obese. There is help, however, and things are not hopeless. Here are some tips to help with your weight-loss journey.

First you must manage your expectations. Losing weight (and keeping it off) is a tough challenge for the majority of people. That is why it is so important to have realistic expectations when getting started. Weight loss is not a race. It is not even a marathon. It is a continuous process. It is doable, however. When you think of all the problems that weight gain causes, you may be surprised to know that just a small reduction, about 5–10 percent of total body weight (typically around ten to twenty pounds), can have a significant impact on your life and help to slow the progression of disease. In diabetic or prediabetic patients, blood-sugar levels improve. Cholesterol levels and blood pressure also decrease thereby reducing the risk of heart disease and stroke. Losing more than 5 percent is a great long-term goal, but focusing on an achievable goal when starting out can have a significant impact on the success of your long-term weight-loss goals.

Second, change your mind-set. Getting into the right mind-set to lose weight is half the battle. It has been said: get your mind in good shape, and then allow your body to follow. It is important to talk to your doctor before beginning any major weight-loss program or exercise routine. Depending on your unique situation, you may have to start your weight-loss efforts with just walking or a mild biking routine until you are able and approved to advance to more strenuous exercises. If this is the case, make sure you are committed to what could be a long and slow journey, especially in the beginning when most people are likely to quit.

Having or getting support is extremely important. If you are going to be successful, it is important to have people in your corner encouraging you to keep going. A great place to start is with close friends and family who will be there to push you forward. If you do not have the support of friends and family, ask your doctor about potential weight-loss support groups you might be able to join. Connecting with people going through the same journey and struggle can increase your chances of success significantly.

Work with your doctor. Losing weight, especially if living with medical problems such as diabetes, requires additional attention to your health. Exercise by itself, with or without weight loss, can improve your body's level of sensitivity to insulin. That is why it is important to keep a record of what you are consuming in terms of calorie intake. Those with diabetes should measure and record blood glucose levels before and after exercise because exercise can lower blood sugar, independent of medications.

While intentional reductions in weight are generally a good thing, unintentional weight loss, especially for people with type 2 diabetes, is not good. When blood-sugar levels are very high, individuals with diabetes will often urinate a lot, which leads to dehydration as a potential reason for weight reduction. Additionally, muscle breakdown occurs when blood sugar is too high, resulting in unhealthy weight loss. These are just a few more reasons to work with your doctor consistently throughout the weight-loss process.

When it comes to weight loss, slow and steady wins the race. A proper diet and exercise plan that will be able to stick to is better than one that you want to quit before you even see results. Remember to have realistic expectations and goals, prepare your mind, build a great support team, and always consult your doctor before getting started

CHAPTER 7

Putting the Pieces Together The Dos and Don'ts of Weight Loss

I keep trying to lose weight...but it keeps finding me!

—UNKNOWN

When most people think of weight-loss or obesity medicine, they think they can take a pill and instantly lose their excess weight, returning them to the way life was prior to their weight gain. We all wish this was true, but when it comes to obesity medication, there are certain rules you should follow to ensure your success. Here are the dos and don'ts of diet medicine:

First, **don't go at it alone**. Dealing with obesity can be a lonely and difficult battle. Not looking or feeling like your self can send you into a spiral of negativity that usually increases the actions that are counterproductive to your weight-loss efforts. You grab the bag of chips, and instead of taking a few out, you sit down with the whole bag. Before you know it, the bag is gone, and you feel even worse about yourself and say, "What the hell, I might as well eat something else." The feeling of helplessness and depression can get worse if you begin taking diet pills and do not see the results you expect as quickly as you expect them. This is usually when people give up and end up returning to their old habits that led to the weight gain in the first place.

Secondly, do find a respected weight-loss specialist. Like most battles in life, having support drastically increases your chances of success. Having a team of weight-loss professionals in your corner that will help you through the mental, physical, and emotional stress of weight loss will help keep you going, especially when you begin to plateau and lose ambition. If you're considering diet medication, you need to go to a respected, local weight-loss specialist. You should go over all your options with the specialist before proceeding with any type of diet medicine.

Third, do not think a diet pill is the magic answer to weight loss. The solution to weight loss is not attributed to any one magical diet pill but attributed to the combination of careful planning, diligent scheduling, and expert guidance. Simply taking the prescription recommended by your weight-loss specialist is not enough. Weight-loss medicines help with suppressing hunger and give you more control over what you eat. You have to include exercise, lifestyle changes (such as removing triggers to overeat), and healthier-eating options.

Fourth, do compliment your diet program and medication with proper exercise and eating habits. A weight-loss prescription is only one aspect of a complete and effective weight-loss program. Working on weight-loss goals requires not only the proper medicine but also the appropriate exercise and eating routines. Diet medication will help control appetite and binge eating, to stop you from continuing to gain weight. However, it's also important to combine your diet medication with complementary exercise and eating habits such as portion control and choosing healthier options in order to achieve maximum results.

Fifth, do not take over-the-counter diet pills. Unproven over-the-counter diet medications are not the answer. In fact, some of the side effects of over-the-counter diet medicines can do more harm than good. Successful weight-loss solutions involve diet prescriptions and programs that are tested and recommended by medical weight-loss professionals. Weight loss does not come from a magic pill, a quick fix, or a supplement sold on an infomercial.

Sixth, do get a custom weight-loss program tailored specifically to your needs. Everyone is different, and every body is different, so make sure the diet medication you take is tailored specifically to you. Make sure your specific needs and symptoms have been looked at thoroughly by a trained endocrinologist or weight-loss specialist. Remember that all medications have side effects, and you do not want to add a medication that will exacerbate a condition you may already have. Conditions such as hypothyroidism, insulin resistance, metabolic syndrome, low estrogen, Cushing's disease, low testosterone, and other hormonal imbalances can all play a factor in your ability to lose weight.

For maximum results, make sure your weight-loss program is comprehensive, starting with proper testing and diagnosis prior to beginning treatment. Have a routine physical exam performed. This includes BMI and/or WC measurement, which helps to characterize obesity and evaluate its complications. Things doctors look for include acanthosis nigricans (darkening of the skin around the neck or under the arms) and multiple skin tags, which are a sign of insulin resistance and prediabetes. Large stretch marks, thinning of the skin can be a sign of excess cortisol (Cushing's syndrome). A large neck may reveal obstructive sleep apnea, and excess hair growth (hirsutism) in women is a sign of polycystic ovarian syndrome. Laboratory evaluation should include tests that evaluate obesity-related conditions. This includes a fasting–blood sugar test, a lipid panel to test for insulin resistance and metabolic syndrome. TSH is the hormone that is used to determine thyroid status. It is the most sensitive for finding problems with the thyroid and is used to rule out hypothy-roidism. Liver function can be tested to evaluate for fatty liver disease and other specific tests, depending on a patient's disease history and medication use. If screening tests are abnormal, and physical exam reveals certain findings, other endocrine or genetic tests may be indicated.

Lastly, do educate yourself. Pick your weight-loss team and start moving forward. It is important to understand that diet medication is only one part of the weight-loss equation. While there is usefulness in the prescribed diet medication, it is important to realize that it is going to take more than just a prescription. Ultimately, the most important factor is whether you are ready to put the pieces of healthy eating, exercise, and lifestyle changes together, and get to work.

CHAPTER 8

Why Medical Weight-Loss Programs Work

Are you tired of following commercial diet and weight-loss programs that promise results but never end up working? You're not alone. Unlike many of those commercial weight-loss services, medical weight-loss programs are different—they actually work.

Like you, we have heard from many patients that have tried dozens of weight-loss gimmicks. They were willing to do anything they had to in order to get back to looking and feeling like themselves again, but no matter how hard they tried, these mass-marketed programs were not able to provide the desired results. If you are tired of trying dozens of heavily marketed programs without results to show for it, then consider a local medical weight-loss program.

A medical weight-loss program offers a customizable approach to weight loss that is closely supervised by a qualified medical team that usually includes a licensed physician, a dietician, and a fitness trainer. Depending on the program and your needs, you may see a variety of other professionals.

Most medical weight-loss programs utilize some or all of the following things, depending on each person's specific health needs and goals:

- Health tests and screenings that identify specific hormonal and metabolic concerns or disorders.
- Prescription weight-loss medications that fit your specific health conditions, lifestyle, and goals.
- An exercise routine that is specific to your physical abilities.
- A diet program that is focused on creating long-term healthy eating habits.
- Support groups and information about making lifestyle changes to reduce behaviors that lead to weight gain.

In direct comparison to gimmicky weight-loss programs and products that you see all over late-night TV, medical weight-loss programs are serious about weight loss. These programs are targeted to your needs and are 100 percent focused on your success, rather than mass sales. If you are serious about considering a medical weight-loss program, here are three reasons the medical approach to weight loss is successful and is usually the best approach for long-term success:

1. It Is a Personalized, Medical Approach to Weight Loss

First it is completely customized to *you*. Unlike typical weight-loss programs that use the same procedures for everyone, medical weight-loss programs treat each patient as an individual, and the specifics of the program will depend on the individual needs and goals of each person. From the beginning, the doctor, dietician, fitness trainer, and all other professionals involved in the program will sit down and discuss your lifestyle, your body, your weight, your habits, and your goals in order to create a plan that helps you succeed in the program and achieve your weight-loss goals.

Some people want to lose a lot of weight so they can look and feel like they did prior to having children, while others just want to lose a few pounds so they are healthier and better able to move around throughout the day. Each person's goals and abilities are different, and a medical weight-loss program will take all of those factors into consideration when creating a customized plan that corresponds to your specific needs and goals.

2. It Is Created and Supervised by Licensed Doctors and Trained Weight-Loss Professionals

When you enroll in a medical weight-loss program, you will not have to worry about not working out enough or whether you are eating the correct foods, or getting the right amount of calories and protein, or about investing your time and resources in other unproven weight-loss remedies.

A professional medical weight-loss program is a supervised program, and every aspect of the program has been carefully planned. This program understands that you are human and bound to make some mistakes. That is why these programs have very realistic weight-loss plans that will enable you to stay on track and help create an environment that motivates you and helps you see long-term results as quickly as possible.

3. It Is Focused on Lifestyle Changes and Sustained Long-Term Success

Unlike other weight-loss programs that usually only provide short-term successes, the goal of a medical weight-loss program is to provide long-term results by changing your body both inside and out. For instance, most people do not realize how big of an impact hormones have on their weight. By simply changing your body's hormonal balance, you could see significant long-term results.

In addition to changing your body, these programs also help you build a lifestyle that supports long-term weight-loss goals. In addition to giving you the tools to lose weight, it will empower you with skills and habits needed to make weight management part of your daily lifestyle, reducing the stress and uncertainty most people have when it comes to their weight. If you are tired of trying new programs, pills, and workout equipment without seeing results, then consider looking into a local medical weight-loss program.

Medical weight-loss programs include various tools to help you achieve the goal of weight loss. First, know your starting point. A tool that helps us figure this out is the body composition scale (BCS). It is a specialized scale that not only measures weight but also gives a breakdown of body composition. This includes not only total body weight but also what percentages are fat, water, and muscle. Based on its calculations, the BCS also provides important information like the basal metabolic rate or BMR. Basal metabolic rate is the measure of how many calories your body burns at rest. These calories are used for essential bodily functions such as breathing and maintaining a normal temperature. When you exercise, walk, move around, or digest food, you use additional calories to perform these functions. With the knowledge of your BMR, you can see how many calories you need to consume each day in order to lose weight. In order to lose one to two pounds per week, you need a five hundred-calorie deficit each day. The BCS provides this information and helps doctors tailor a meal plan specific to you. People who are larger burn more calories and have higher calorie intake than smaller people. However, as you lose weight, gain muscle, and become more active, your BMR changes, and things evolve. Your caloric needs change and decrease. This decrease varies per person, and the body adapts to weight loss with reduced energy expenditure (Ryan and Wyatt 2015). This reduction in energy output is disproportionate to weight reduction. For example, Mr. Smith weighs 220 pounds, and at that weight, he needs twenty-two hundred calories per day. His friend Mr. Jones weighs two hundred pounds and needs two thousand calories per day. Mr. Smith works out, cuts down on some junk food, and loses twenty pounds and now weighs two hundred pounds. His caloric requirements decreased, so he now only needs 1,830 calories per day to maintain his weight (Schwartz and Doucet 2010). You can see, despite being the same weight, Mr. Smith requires less calories in order to maintain his weight. Because of the body's adaptation and resistance to weight loss, one has to change his or her approach to how much they eat or burn off through exercise in order to maintain or continue to lose weight. To put it simply, the body wants to stay at its current weight. When you try to change with cutting calories and food intake, hormone levels change, hunger increases, and the number of calories needed decreases. When these changes happen, you may find that even though you eat the same amount, you can gain weight. Tools like the BCS help you to see where you are baseline as far as BMR is concerned and give you an idea of how many calories you need to either decrease your intake or burn off in order to lose weight. Once you have lost weight, it can help you to see the changes not only in body-fat percentage but also in your new BMR. This gives you a better idea of where you have to go from there to continue to get to your goal.

Figures 7 and 8 are examples of a female patient's BCS results before and after weight loss, and figures 9 and 10 are a male patient's BCS results. Identifying information has been removed. Notice the change after weight loss not only in the weight and fat percentages but also in the metabolic rate.

```
B O D Y   C O M P O S I T I O N   R E P O R T      Date: 10/26/2015
─────────────────────────────────────────────────────────────────

Name: ___

Gender: F          Hgt: 5' 10.0"           Age:  57    BioAge: 66
                        177 cm


Prepared By: 7
─────────────────────────────────────────────────────────────────
              Current Body Weight      242.3 Lbs
                                       109.9 Kg

              Total Body Fat            42.1 %
                                       101.3 Lbs
                                        45.9 Kg

              Visceral Fat                13

              Fat-Free Mass             57.8 %
                                       138.9 Lbs
                                        63.0 Kg

              Total Body Water          43.4 %
                                       104.3 Lbs
                                        47.3 Kg

              Muscle-Mass
                                        34.6 Lbs
                                        15.7 Kg

              Body Mass Index           34.7
```

Body Fat Total	% Body Water Norms	Body Fat Ranges	
13-19	64-56%		
20-29	55-46%	Athletic	13-20%
30-39	45-40%	Normal	21-27%
40+	39-32%	Sedentary	28%+

```
Basal Metabolic Rate 1753 Calories/Day

      Activity Level    Daily Caloric Needs
      ──────────────────────────────────────
      Very Light        1929   Calories/Day
      Light             2104   Calories/Day
      Moderate          2279   Calories/Day
      Heavy             2630   Calories/Day
      Very Heavy        2981   Calories/Day
```

Valhalla Scientific, • 121/1 Ruddman Road, Poway, CA 92064
658.457.5575 • www.cloud.compnrole.com   For sales or services call 800.548.9808

Figure 7: Body Composition for female before weight loss

```
BODY  COMPOSITION  REPORT    Date: 02/26/2016

Name: ___                    _____

Gender: F        Hgt: 5' 11.0"        Age:  58    BioAge: 64
                      180 cm      Ohms:  620


Prepared By: _____  _____

        Current Body Weight        221.6 Lbs
                                    100.5 Kg

        Total Body Fat             39.0 %
                                    85.6 Lbs
                                    38.8 Kg

        Visceral Fat               11

        Fat-Free Mass              60.9 %
                                   133.9 Lbs
                                    60.7 Kg

        Total Body Water          -44.9 %
                                    98.8 Lbs
                                    44.8 Kg

        Muscle-Mass                 35.1 Lbs
                                    15.9 Kg

        Body Mass Index            30.7
```

Body Fat Total	% Body Water Norms	Body Fat Ranges	
13-19	64-56%		
20-29	55-46%	Athletic	13-20%
30-39	45-40%	Normal	21-27%
40+	39-32%	Sedentary	28%+

```
Basal Metabolic Rate 1673 Calories/Day

Activity Level    Daily Caloric Needs

    Very Light      1841    Calories/Day
    Light           2008    Calories/Day
    Moderate        2175    Calories/Day
    Heavy           2510    Calories/Day
    Very Heavy      2845    Calories/Day
```

Figure 8: Body Composition for female patient after weight loss

```
B O D Y   C O M P O S I T I O N   R E P O R T      Date: 9-24-15


Name:
Gender: M          Hgt: 5' 11.0"          Age: 56    BioAge: 73
                        180 cm


Prepared By: 7

          Current Body Weight      307.8 Lbs
                                    139.6 Kg

          Total Body Fat            40.2 %
                                    122.9 Lbs
                                     55.7 Kg

          Visceral Fat                32

          Fat-Free Mass             59.7 %
                                    182.7 Lbs
                                     82.9 Kg

          Total Body Water          40.7 %
                                    124.6 Lbs
                                     56.5 Kg

          Muscle-Mass
                                     58.0 Lbs
                                     26.3 Kg

          Body Mass Index           42.8
```

Body Fat Total	% Body Water Norms	Body Fat Ranges	
5-12	72-68%		
13-19	67-60%	Athletic	6-13%
20-29	59-54%	Normal	14-19%
30-45	53-40%	Sedentary	20%+

```
Basal Metabolic Rate 2240 Calories/Day

   Activity Level   Daily Caloric Needs

   Very Light      2688    Calories/Day
   Light           3136    Calories/Day
   Moderate        3360    Calories/Day
   Heavy           3808    Calories/Day
   Very Heavy      4256    Calories/Day
```

Figure 9: Body Composition for male patient before weight loss

BODY COMPOSITION REPORT   Date: 01/29/14

Name: _____

Gender: M   Hgt: 5' 11.0"   Age: 56   BioAge: 65
                      180 cm   Ohms: 536

Prepared By: _____

Current Body Weight	244.3 Lbs 110.8 Kg
Total Body Fat	32.7 % 79.3 Lbs 36.0 Kg
Visceral Fat	21
Fat-Free Mass	67.2 % 162.9 Lbs 73.8 Kg
Total Body Water	48.2 % 116.8 Lbs 53.0 Kg
Muscle-Mass	46.0 Lbs 20.8 Kg
Body Mass Index	33.9

Body Fat Total	% Body Water Norms	Body Fat Ranges	
5-12	72-68%		
13-19	67-60%	Athletic	6-13%
20-29	59-54%	Normal	14-19%
30-45	53-40%	Sedentary	20%+

Basal Metabolic Rate 1952 Calories/Day

Activity Level	Daily Caloric Needs	
Very Light	2342	Calories/Day
Light	2733	Calories/Day
Moderate	2928	Calories/Day
Heavy	3319	Calories/Day
Very Heavy	3709	Calories/Day

BODY COMP SCALE

Valhalla Scientific • 12127 Kirkham Road, Poway, CA 92064   5   For sales or services call 800.548.980
818.457.5576 • www.bodycompscale.com

Figure 10: Body Composition for male patient after weight loss

Meal-replacement programs are also optional treatments that can aid in weight loss. There are a variety of programs available. They work because they take the guesswork out of eating by providing low-calorie, high-nutrition alternatives to meals. Meal replacement is done for a finite time, and regular food is later reintroduced into the diet.

The basic rule of weight loss is a balance between calories in and calories out. When you eat, you consume energy or calories. If you use or burn less calories than you intake, you have a positive energy balance, and the excess energy is stored as fat. When you burn off or expend more calories than you intake, you have a negative energy balance, and the body then converts the stored body fat into energy, and you lose weight. In any instance of weight loss, you must have a negative energy balance in order to lose weight. Meal-replacement programs such as OPTIFAST allow you to do this by giving you portion-controlled products with a set number of calories. It helps you to have tight control over your caloric intake without measuring out your food and counting calories. This makes it easier to consume fewer calories over a longer period of time. Using meal-replacement products such as shakes, protein bars, and soups takes the guesswork out of your meal planning. This allows you to focus on other things, such as exercise, being more active, and making lifestyle changes (such as healthier food choices and developing a support system to help you during difficult times—holidays or birthdays—when people tend to fall back into old habits).

Meal-replacement programs offer low-calorie options that are low in fat, low in carbohydrates, and high in quality protein. This is important because lowering fat helps decrease both caloric intake and cholesterol levels. Meal-replacement products do have some fat, however, which is important for absorption of fat-soluble vitamins A, D, E, and K. Carbohydrates are used by most tissues in the body for fuel and are necessary for functioning of the brain and central nervous system. Your brain can only use glucose as fuel, so if the glucose around is not enough, you break down muscle in order to form glucose. This is why people on low-calorie diets and low-carb diets often lose not only fat but also muscle. Because of the balance of nutrients, glucose, protein, and a necessary amount of fat, meal-replacement products such as shakes, protein bars, and soups help you to lower calories without missing out on necessary nutrients. What about vitamins and minerals? These are included in the products as well so that you get total nutrition when products are taken as prescribed.

After using meal-replacement products for a period of time and under the supervision of a physician, you gradually return to self-prepared food. This helps you to slowly work on controlling your calorie intake on your own and develops the skills to make and choose healthier meal options. Your doctor, personal trainer, and weight-loss program are all there to help you throughout the process to first reach your weight-loss goal and then maintain your weight and deal with fluctuations in weight that will occur. Remember this is a long-term process, and you need both short-term and long-term goals and plans to succeed.

Tips to using a meal-replacement program successfully include the following:

- Remember it is more like a marathon than a sprint, so take things one day at a time. The weight gain did not happen overnight, and it will not go away overnight.
- You can always get back on track if you falter, sneak a treat, or have a big meal. You do not have to wait until the next day or week. Try not to beat yourself up, and just resolve to achieve your goals.
- Plan ahead. Take your products with you to work, when going out shopping, or when away from home so you are less likely to be tempted to grab just anything.
- Record your food intake and physical activity. This helps you to be accountable and see exactly what you are doing.

- Make sure you drink plenty of water. This helps to fill you up when you feel hungry.
- Keep active. This helps to keep your mind off of food.
- Increase your physical activity as tolerated.
- Reward yourself with something other than food.
- Discuss with family and friends how they can be supportive and help you throughout your weight-loss journey. Give specifics, such as not eating junk food around you, joining you on a walk, or helping to go grocery shopping or cooking.
- Lastly follow your diet prescription.

As you decrease calories, even with meal replacement, you can develop symptoms. Some of the changes are due to changes in your body, and some are psychological, especially in the first few weeks of starting a program. If you develop any problems, discuss them with your doctor right away. Fatigue is the most common problem. When you start to consume less calories than your body is used to, you may feel weak and tired. Try to get plenty of rest, and do not overexert yourself with exercise. When starting out, do moderate activities that do not leave you feeling drained and exhausted. Drinking water is important because not doing so can result in dizziness, dry mouth, or headaches. Your body loses water and salt during weight loss and exercise, so make sure you replace it with fluid intake, and do not skip meals—this can lead to headaches and feelings of weakness. If you are used to eating high-calorie, sugary, and salty foods, you can develop cravings for them when they are removed. Be mindful that these cravings are temporary. Distract yourself with other activities or thoughts. Most importantly do not give up on your program. As you continue to go along and start to lose weight, you will feel better, have more energy, and be able to move better. Just remember that you are on the way to a new and improved you.

CHAPTER 9

How Exercise Improves Weight Loss

The goal of this chapter is to clarify a few things about exercise. Exercise in conjunction with diet is critical to weight loss and weight maintenance, not only for obese people but also for the general population. Although it can be challenging for obese and overweight patients to transition to a healthy lifestyle, the physical and emotional benefits of a regular exercise program make it worth the effort.

How does exercise improve weight loss? First of all, when we talk about exercise, that does not necessarily mean going to the gym, giving money away for a gym membership you do not use, or buying exercise equipment, such as a treadmill, and then using it as a clothes hanger. Any kind of physical activity that gets your heart rate up can be an exercise. The trick is to find an activity that you enjoy and will continue with over time. The benefits of exercise are tremendous.

Regular exercise helps to lower blood pressure and improve choles-terol numbers in addition to improving insulin sensitivity and blood-sugar control. Exercise helps to increase stamina, keep bones strong, and promotes improvement in balance, depending on the type of activity. Exercise also has a huge impact on one's mental outlook and makes you feel better overall.

As mentioned earlier, genes such as the FTO gene contribute to obesity and weight gain. That does not mean that all is lost to the whim of Mother Nature. A recent article in *Nature* revealed that exer-cise can decrease the impact of the obesity gene FTO on weight gain and BMI. The authors of the article demonstrated that people with high-risk obesity genes who exercised vigorously for an hour per week decreased the weight gain by 36–75 percent, compared to those who had low level of physical activity (Reddon et al. 2016).

There are different types of exercises. Aerobic exercise is the most commonly studied exercise and has the most benefit on various met-abolic factors and weight loss. Aerobic exercise is that which increases heart rate and strengthens the heart and lungs. Any physical activity is good, and exercises that have less impact on the joints are less likely to cause pain and injury. Aerobic exercises include things like walking, running, bike riding, skating, use of the elliptical machine, and swim-ming. Many patients can tolerate exercises such as walking or bike riding, but for those with joint problems, swimming is a great exercise. For patients who have not done any exercise, it is good for them to start slow and work their way up so that they can keep up and not get discouraged. Walking is the easiest way for most people to get started with an exercise program, according to John P. Higgins and Christopher Higgins of the Cleveland Clinic. Walking is safe, accessible, and requires no equipment. High-intensity interval training, or HIIT, involves short spurts of vigorous activity alternating with periods of recovery. Aerobic exercise is the foundation for weight loss because it increases the heart rate and oxygenation in the lungs. Over time, one should vary the type of exercise to use different muscle groups in order to decrease the risk of injury or overuse of one muscle or joint group (Higgins and Higgins 2016). Resistance training, flexibility, and balance exercises also provide valuable improvements and changes to the body. Resistance exercises that are progressive are easier for obese patients. They allow patients to work with other more active people and can help improve mood and positivity after completing sets of exercise. Resistance/strength exercises not only use weights or body weight to increase muscle strength but can also lead to fat reduction. The reduction of fat improves insulin resistance in overweight and obese people. Resistance training works by causing a breakdown or tear in the muscle, and as the muscle is repaired, it becomes stronger.

Due to the remodeling of muscle tissue, resistance exercises should be done on nonconsecutive days to allow the muscles to heal in between exercise.

Flexibility and balance exercises help to improve the movement of muscles and joints and also improve stability. Poor balance and flexibility is associated with more injuries, accidents, and falls during daily normal activities. An excellent way to improve both is with yoga. Yoga improves not only flexibility and balance but also strength. These combined may help to decrease stress and improve blood pressure, cholesterol and insulin resistance, as well as the ability to exercise.

For people who are extremely obese, low-impact exercises such as walking, bike riding, and water aerobics are easier to manage and still effective as long as they are done on a consistent basis. Patients who have not done any regular exercise and want to start an exercise program should be evaluated by his or her physician. Choosing any exercise that gets you moving and that you enjoy is a good idea. According to the American Colleges of Sports Medicine (ACSM), it is recommended that one combine aerobic and resistance exercise into an exercise program (Garber et al. 2011; Donnelly et al. 2009). This has been shown to lead to a decrease in obesity in the abdomen, which is the problem area for most people. Recommendations for weight loss and exercise are to exercise most days of the week at low to moderate intensity. Low intensity is when you feel your heart rate increase but can still carry on a conversation. Moderate intensity is when the heart rate increases, but you can answer only in short sentences. The goal is 150 minutes of aerobic exercise per week. Resistance training is recommended two to three times per week on nonconsecutive days. You want to do exercises that work eight to ten muscle groups per session, doing two to four sets of ten repetitions for each muscle group. Stretching for flexibility should include a stretch of a muscle for at least fifteen seconds and should be done two to four times per week. Just remember that, when starting any exercise program, if you are not used to exercising, start slowly at low impact, and work your way up to increased intensity, time spent exercising, and frequency of exercise.

Often people who are obese do not do well when told to exercise. It is difficult to start an exercise program due to fatigue, lack of support, lack of time, or lack of motivation. The weight did not come on overnight, and it is not going to go away quickly, either. Set simple, achievable goals. In an article on exercise in the *CCJM* (Higgins and Higgins 2016), SMART goals are mentioned. Goals that are "**s**pecific, **m**easurable, **a**ttainable, **r**ealistic and **t**imely should be set to sustain the self-discipline required" to make life-style changes and reach weight-loss goals. Today there are numerous tools that help you to reach these goals. Smartphone apps help to remind you to exercise and can track your level of activity. In the beginning of your weight-loss journey, a personal trainer is an important tool because he or she will keep you accountable. All in all, physical activity and exercise of any type is beneficial, but as with life, variety is the spice that makes things better.

So what is the best exercise for weight loss? Any structured, repetitive, body motion (exercise) that you will do on a regular basis. While research shows aerobic exercise is the best for weight loss it is important to vary your routine and also to incorporate strength training to maintain muscle mass. This is important because after intense exercise muscle burns more calories than fat tissue and also continues to burn calories after exercise. This is known as the after-burn or post-exercise calorie burn. This calorie burn is the result of muscle repairing itself from microscopic tears and damage after strenuous exercise. An example of an exercise plan includes both cardiovascular (cardio) exercise alternating with strength training. Exercise should be done most days of the week, four-six days per week, if weight loss is the goal.

Workout- Schedule	Type of Exercise	Duration of Time
Monday	Cardio	60 minutes
Tuesday	Cardio warm-up 15 minutes Strength training 45 minutes	60 minutes
Wednesday	Cardio	60 minutes
Thursday	Cardio warm-up 15 minutes Strength training 45 minutes	60 m
Friday	Cardio	60 minutes
Saturday	Rest day or stretching/yoga	30-60 minutes
Sunday	Rest day	

Examples of cardio exercise include: running/jogging, walking, biking, swimming, dancing, stair climbing, elliptical machine, step aerobics, and cardio-kickboxing. Cardiovascular exercise works not only the arms and legs but also the heart. Your heart rate should increase during exercise and you should feel like you are working. Aim for moderate intensity exercise with heart rate in the 110-130 range. More vigorous intensity is a heart in the 140-160 range. Do not start with vigorous intensity in an attempt to lose weight faster especially if you are new to exercise. Start at a comfortable pace and each week try to increase the intensity as tolerated until you get to moderate intensity. Always make sure you consult your physician when you are starting and new work out program.

Strength training includes the use of weights and body-weight exercises such as push-ups, pull-ups, plank holds, squats and lunges with-or without weights. The goal of strength training is to increase strength and muscle endurance. Alternate the muscle groups worked on days of that you do strength training to reduce overuse of one or two muscle groups.   For instance, using the example exercise plan you would do upper body exercises on Tuesday and lower body on Thursday.   Do eight to ten repetitions for three sets for each exercise you do. The weight should be heavy enough that the last 3 repetitions are hard. If you can easily do 10 repetitions then you need to increase the weight.

Remember your body is changing. You want it to change and in order to do that you have to challenge yourself. Exercise is not easy but when done consistently it is rewarding. The rewards include weight loss, increased strength, endurance, energy and more restful sleep. This is in addition to all the health benefits we have mentioned like decreased blood sugar, improved blood pressure, cholesterol and decreased risk of long-term serious disease.

Although exercise can be tough it does not need to break the bank. Exercise can be done at home or outdoors. Many websites offer numerous exercise videos to guide your workout. There are also variations on traditional exercises. For the upper body consider push-ups. This works the arms, shoulders and chest. While the traditional push-up is both hands on the floor, body position starting in a plank then dropping down to the ground and pushing back up this can be modified to fit you. One modification is to start on the knees in a plank position, lower the body, then push the chest up off the ground. What if that is too hard? Find a stable chair in the house. Push the chair against the wall to avoid sliding. Start with your hands on the edge of the chair and you in an upright position on the knees. Then lower your body down towards the chair and push- back up. That is one repetition. Can't get on your knees? Well push off the wall. Place both feet together on the floor, lean into the wall elbows bent and push back until the elbows are extended. Repeat that motion for a count of ten. That is one set. Lower body exercises include squats, lunges, hip raises. If you have joint problems, no sweat, you can still work your legs. First modification is to not squat down or lunge as low or deep. If that is not possible sit in a chair and raise your leg straight until it is parallel with the chair for a count of ten. To work the opposite muscles, stand with your hands on a chair in front of you for balance and curl your leg back up towards the buttocks. This is a hamstring curl. Calf raises work the lower leg. They can be performed standing alone or holding onto the wall or a chair for balance. Start with your feet parallel and rise up onto your toes then lower back down to your heels. Repeat ten times fast then ten times slow for set of three each.

If you want to make exercise harder but you don't have weights milk jugs, water jugs, and canned good can substitute for weights. These items can be used for bicep curls, overhead press, tricep extensions, front and side arm raises and chest press. For the lower body these items can used when doing squats, lunges and calf raises. In the gym these exercises are done with machines or free weights like dumbbells or kettlebells. Remember any exercise can be modified to fit your current level of fitness. Over time as exercises become easier and you become stronger you have to increase the weight and vary your routine to continue your progess.

CHAPTER 10

Adjunctive Therapy and Technology

There are many tools and ways to help you combat stress that leads to altered hormone levels, emotional eating, fatigue, and depression. These include adjunct therapies that help with fitness, relaxation, and muscle soreness. Exercise is always recommended for weight loss and helps to burn those extra calories. However, when people do not see instant results or, despite exercise, the body's adaptation response kicks in and counters weight loss or leads to weight regain, people become discouraged and often quit. Working with a trainer or at least a workout partner can help to motivate you. As physicians we recommend that our patients find an activity that they like because they are more likely to continue it. Try new things such as different classes. Venture outdoors when the weather allows for biking, hiking, or other outdoor activities and sports. For those with joint problems, swimming or water aerobics is a good exercise because you do not get the hard impact on the joints that comes with running, jogging, jumping, and other high-impact activities. You want to work different muscle groups so that your body does not get used to doing the same old thing. Cardio exercise is important but so is building strength and muscle. It helps with balance and toning, and the muscle burns more calories, even at rest, than fat tissue. A fitness trainer can help you develop a program to fit your needs. But what about the soreness and aches that come with starting exercise or too much exercise? Consider massage therapy, yoga, and stretching. These things help to soothe and lengthen those tight, tired muscles. They also help you to relax. Consider yoga once a week; it not only helps to stretch muscles, but it also builds strength. Massages can be costly, but consider treating yourself once a month or once every few months. Ask yourself what will benefit you more in the long run: treating yourself to a large meal, dessert, and drinks which you will end up regretting or something that will help you relax and improve your health and decrease the risk of health problems in the future. Furthermore consider music therapy. It has been said that music is the universal language. Whether you are young or old, there is music that soothes you, helps you to relax, and moves you. Unwind by listening to your favorite tune. Listen to something energizing to get you through your workout, and later relax to some mellow music. Last but not least, get a good night's sleep on a consistent basis. Sleep is important. Several studies have shown a relationship between lack of sleep and weight gain/obesity. The number of people with short sleep (five to six hours per night) who are overweight appears to be increasing over the past thirty-two years (Girardin et al. 2014). Sleep is an important regulator of hormonal function and glucose (sugar) metabolism. Several studies have shown that sleep loss leads to changes in metabolic and endocrine function, such as "decreased glucose tolerance, decreased insulin sensitivity, increased evening concentrations of cortisol, increased levels of ghrelin, decreased levels of leptin, and increased hunger and appetite" (Beccuti and Pannain 2011).

When you look at maps of sleep deprivation and obesity in the United States, there appears to be a correlation. States with the most obesity are also ones with the most sleep deprivation.

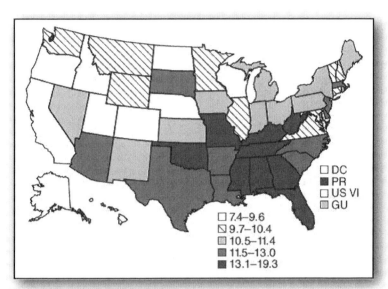

Figure 11. Map of sleep insufficiency.

The map below depicts age-adjusted* percentage of adults who reported thirty days of insufficient rest
or sleep† during the preceding thirty days. Data is from the 2008 Behavioral Risk Factor Surveillance
System, United States.‡

* Age adjusted to 2000 projected US population.

† Determined by response to the question, "During the past thirty days, for about how many days have you felt you did not get enough rest or sleep?"

‡ Includes the fifty states, District of Columbia, Guam, Puerto Rico, and US Virgin Islands,
http://www.cdc.gov/sleep/data_statistics.html.

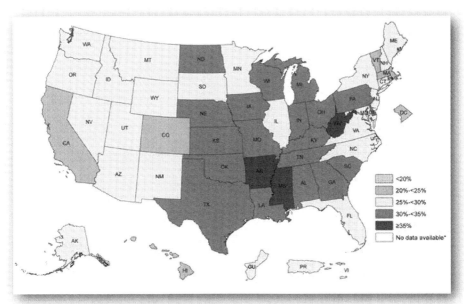

Figure 12. Prevalence of self-reported obesity among
US adults by state and territory, BRFSS, 2014.

Prevalence estimates reflect BRFSS methodological changes started in 2011.
These estimates should not be compared to prevalence estimates before 2011.

Source: Behavioral Risk Factor Surveillance System, CDC, http://www.cdc.gov/
obesity/data/prevalence-maps.html.

Technology has been both a help and a hindrance to us. The automobile allowed us to travel farther quicker but it also decreased people's need to walk and move. Drive-thru fast food places made quick high calorie meals easily available. So instead of burning calories from your hamburger while walking home those same calories you consume get stored as fat on the comfortable drive back home. Microwave ovens help to warm and cook food quickly but lead the way to more calorie-dense but nutrient-poor meals and snacks like tv dinners and microwave popcorn. Remote controls removed the need to get up to change the channel on the television. Our phones and tablets allow us to access to an enormous amount of information and connect to others like never before but they also keep us from sleep which we talk, read, play games and connect on social media. Not to mention the light from various devices which is shown to decrease sleep quality and duration. Nowadays children do not go outside to play. Instead they are glued to tablet devices or their parent's phone watching videos and playing games.

Despite these facts new technology is available to get us moving again. Activity trackers, specialized watches and apps are available to encourage movement, track food and calorie intake and help you stick to weight loss goals. The most common trackers are Fitbit, Jawbone, Nike Fuelband and Lark.

Fitbit

Fitbit offers a wide variety of devices that either clip to the clothes or are worn on the wrist. This tracker tracks steps, calories burned, sleep duration and quality and through mobile app helps you keep track of your fitness goals daily.

Jawbone

Jawbone is a sophisticated bracelet that tracks your activity, food intake, sleep and mood.

Nike FuelBand

Nike FuelBand is also a wrist band that tracks calories and activities. A mobile app is also available to monitor your fitness goals.

Lark

Lark includes both night and daytime wristbands. Its app allows you to monitor food intake, exercise, calories ingested and sleep as well. This information allows you to see exactly what you are doing and make adjustments were needed.

When it comes to health apps there are approximately forty-thousand apps available. Some are free and others cost a fee. The market for health apps is growing rapidly. Theses apps provide information that would otherwise be assumed leading to over estimation of exercise and under estimation of food intake. They help hold people accountable to what they are doing. When someone is watching, even a machine people are more likely to stick to their goals. Some of the most popular weight loss apps include MyFitnessPal, Fitness Builder, Nike+ Running, RunKeeper and Endomondo Sport Tracker.

MyFitnessPal

This app allows you to track your activity and food intake using a food diary and activity log. It has an extensive food database and you can find calorie information for almost anything, about 1 million food items. There is also the option to add your own foods and recipes. This app is easy to use and allows you to see the breakdown of your nutritional intake by telling you the grams of carbohydrates, fat and protein you have consumed.

Fitness Builder

This is one of the most useful apps for tracking exercise. Just as MyFitnessPal has an extensive food database Fitness Builder has an extensive exercise database. It contains exercise images, videos as well as access to a live personal trainer. All types of exercises are included along with calculator and tracking features.

Nike+Running and RunKeeper

These apps are perfect for those who love to run or jog. They allow you to map your run as well as monitor distance, speed and the number of calories burned. They track your location when running using GPS and allow sharing of your information and goals with your social networks. In addition RunKeeper allows you to set goals, compare activity stats with others and provides training plans and voice coaching.

Endomondo Sports Tracker

This app not only lets you track your heart rate, calorie intake, speed, distance but has built in GPS to track your route on a map. With the input of goals an audio coach gives you feed back while exercising to keep you motivated. It is like having your own personal trainer in your pocket. Sharing with friend and tracking the workouts of others in real-time is also available.

There are also a number of other useful apps you may not have heard of but you should check out.

GAIN Fitness

Gain Fitness has digital personal trainers and creates personalized workout routines based on your fitness level and goals.

Gympact

Gympact helps you reach goals by providing a monetary incentive. First you set your goals like how many times you will go to the gym per week. Then you set a monetary amount you will be willing to pay if you do not reach that goal. If you reach your target you earn a cash reward. If you do not you then you "contribute" your money to a communit pot that pays others who reach their goals.

JEFIT

This app lets you expand your workout by providing exercises and routines used by bodybuilders. You can search by muscle group and by the equipment you have available.

Keas

This app provides a platform to create a healthier work environment. It allows people to form teams and compete with coworkers to lose weight and become healthier. Cash or other prizes are offered by employers to make the experience competitive and worthwhile.

MapMyFitness

MapMyFitness uses a combination of websites and apps to track not only outdoor activities but also nutritional information. It also provides up to date weather, traffic and information about safer routes that impact your outdoor workouts. You can also compare you progress with friends.

Lift

Lift provides a unique function in that it allows incorporate almost any goal you want to achieve weight loss, become healthy or improve productivity. It allows you to break down your goals into smaller more achievable habits and track whether you achieve them.

Pocket Yoga

This app is for anyone looking to start or continue their yoga practice at home. It offers voice instruction and visual guides for developing yoga skills

Retrofit

This app combines information from various sources like Fitbit tracker and wireless scales. What makes this app unique is that it uses Skype along with information from other sources and to develop personalized video sessions via Skype with fitness and wellness experts to help you change habits and achieve your goals.

Skimble Workout Trainer

With this app you have access to hundreds of workouts both audio and visual to help you exercise with or without equipment.

CHAPTER 11

Why Medications?

Often people are looking for a quick fix to lose weight. This is for various reasons. They want to look good for the summer, lose weight for a wedding or vacation, or to improve their health. Whatever the reason people want to shed extra pounds, we should all realize that over-the-counter (OTC) pills and fad diets, which are a quick fix, often fail. They can be dangerous, and if they do work, the weight loss often is regained quickly. So what works? You might think I do not want to depend on a pill to lose weight or become dependent on medication. One thing you have to remember is that weight gain does not occur overnight. For most people, it occurs gradually over years. Those extra sweets and big plates around the holidays add extra pounds that we plan to shed but never do. Then vacation comes, and you want to relax with alcoholic drinks, and eat as much as you please. Those five to ten pounds gained add up over the years, and when you look back five to ten years later, you have gained fifty pounds. Because weight gain did not occur overnight, it is not going to disappear overnight. Obesity is a chronic disease with various factors from genetics to stress, hormone changes, and adaptations that signal you to eat. Readily available foods high in sugar and salt stimulate the brain's reward system and lead to cravings. Cutting back works to a point, but then you cannot fight the hunger or cravings. Exercise helps you to burn off the excess calories but can make you feel hungrier afterward, leading to consuming calories that you just burned. US Food and Drug Administration (FDA)–approved medications can help to counteract these problems. Just like any disease, there are certain lifestyle changes you can make that take you so far, and then there are medications to help you control and treat the disease. Obesity is no exception. Medications may need to be used long-term, but often these medicines are not covered by health insurance.

In the past four to five years, the FDA-approved options for weight loss have expanded greatly. Prior to 2012, phentermine (which was first approved in 1959) and orlistat (approved in 1999) were the only two options available for weight loss. Before that, various medicines had been tried but removed from the market due to serious side effects. This has made people hesitant to consider medications with potentially small benefits but big side effects. Now four new agents have been approved by the FDA and offer safer options. Before new medications are approved, they have to undergo rigorous testing and show that they do not cause increased risk of heart attack or stroke.

Which medication is best depends on the person. People respond differently to each medication. In general one can expect 5–12 percent weight loss with medications in addition to lifestyle changes. All obesity medications are contraindicated during pregnancy. Each medication available works to suppress appetite and/or increase fullness. However, they work on different receptors; therefore they have different side effects. Deciding which medication is best for you should involve a discussion between you and your doctor and depends on your circumstances. Any prescribed weight-loss medication should be taken while under the supervision of a licensed physician.

Weight-loss medication should be considered when a person with a BMI between 25 and 26.9 has not had much weight-loss success with diet, exercise, and lifestyle changes. Those with BMI between 27 and 29.9 should also make lifestyle changes, but if they also have obesity-related complications such as diabetes, high blood pressure, or high cholesterol, then medication should be considered. Those with BMI >30 should be treated with medication as well as diet and exercise.

Phentermine

Phentermine is a stimulant medication that suppresses the appetite. It is approved for short-term use for weight loss in adults with BMI >30 or those with BMI >27 and health problems such as diabetes. It is FDA-approved for three months' use only but can be taken intermittently. It ranges from doses of 15 mg to 37.5 mg daily. It is recommended that it be taken in the morning to curb the appetite during the day and because it can lead to insomnia due to the stimulant effects. Its use is limited to twelve weeks of continuous use. Patients can develop a decreased efficacy with longer continuous use. Phentermine is not safe for use during pregnancy. It should not be used while nursing or taking monoamine oxidase inhibitor (MAOI) medications. Patients with glaucoma, current hyperthyroidism, and history of drug abuse should not use this. Relative contraindications include tachycardia (rapid heartbeat), hypertension, and heart disease or arrhythmia (irregular heartbeat) (Kahan 2015).

Orlistat

Orlistat is a medication that blocks the absorption of fat from food so that it is not digested. It is approved for long-term use and leads to an average weight loss of 4–6 percent. Side effects include oily/greasy stools, diarrhea, and bowel-movement urgency. However, it has the least side effects or interactions with other medications.

Phentermine/Topiramate ER

Phentermine/topiramate extended-release formulation is a combination of the weight-loss medicine phentermine and topiramate, a seizure medicine. It produces more weight loss at lower doses than either medicine alone. It is approved for long-term use. There are multiple dosages available that range from 7.5/46 mg to 15/92 mg phentermine/topiramate. Weight loss is 8–10 percent and averages between twenty and twenty-four pounds in six months, with the weight loss being maintained for one to two years. Side effects are similar to that of phentermine, with the additional side effects of numbness/tingling, changes in mental function, risk of seizure when discontinued abruptly, and a rare form of glaucoma. Topiramate causes birth defects, and any woman on the medication should have a pregnancy test prior to starting the medication. **Lorcaserin**

Lorcaserin is a serotonin 2c receptor agonist that is specific to the brain and not to receptors on the heart, like previous weight-loss medications. The activation of heart receptors is what caused serious side effects like heart-valve disease and increased risk of heart attack in weight loss medications removed from the market. Lorcaserin works on the brain to increase satiety. It is dosed at 10 mg twice daily and is approved for long-term use. Weight loss is 4–6 percent, similar to orlistat or phentermine. Side effects include headache, dizziness, and nausea. It can worsen depression in people who are prone to or are currently suffering from depression.

Naltrexone SR/Bupropion SR

Naltrexone/bupropion is a combination of naltrexone, an opioid pain-medicine antagonist, and bupropion, an antidepressant. Weight loss is about 6–8 percent or eight to fifteen pounds. It can lead to high blood pressure and rapid pulse. Other side effects include headache, constipation or diarrhea, dry mouth, and anxiety and worsening depression.

Liraglutide

Liraglutide is a glucagon-like peptide-1 (GLP-1) agonist. GLP-1 agonists are approved for diabetes treatment, but in December of 2014, liraglutide was approved at 3 mg dose for weight loss. GLP-1 has various actions of which include decreased hunger and early satiety. Weight loss ranges from 6 to 8 percent (eight to eighteen pounds), and the effects last for at least two years. Side effects include nausea, diarrhea, vomiting, and (rarely) pancreatitis.

Weight-loss medications help people lose weight when added to diet and exercise. One should not depend on weight-loss medications alone. Most chronic diseases need combination therapy. Obesity is no different. Lifestyle changes plus medications have been shown to be better than either alone (Wadden et al. 2005). Medications have been shown to improve several health and heart-disease risk factors to varying degrees. Orlistat leads to decreases in blood sugar and blood pressure. Lorcaserin has been shown to help decrease blood pressure and total cholesterol with weight loss, and phentermine/topiramate showed similar effects. Patients on naltrexone/bupropion and liraglutide showed reductions in blood pressure, blood sugar, and LDL (bad cholesterol). This is important because obesity is linked to the development of diabetes, heart disease, and high cholesterol. When uncontrolled over time, these risk factors lead to increased mortality. There is variability in the response to treatment among the different medications, but with more options available, we can now individualize treatment. Medications are important for short-term weight loss and long-term weight maintenance. Medication helps control hunger and, along with diet and exercise, can have a significant impact on one's health. Although weight loss, not health, may be the primary focus, there are additional benefits to even a small amount of weight loss.

CHAPTER 12

Weight-Loss Surgery and Weight-loss Procedures

O besity treatment is like a pyramid. The large base consists of diet, portion control, exercise, and behavioral changes. This applies to everyone. On the next level, medications are added for those who are moderately obese. Finally, at the top of the pyramid, surgery is recommended for those with severe obesity.

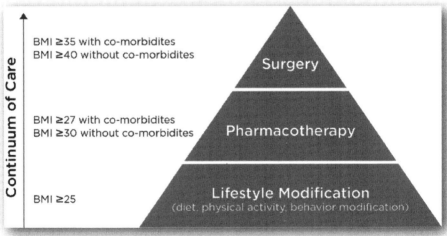

Figure 13. Treatment pyramid for obesity.

Bariatric (weight loss) surgery is a valuable tool for weight loss and long-term success. It is reserved for people with severe obesity and BMI >40 or BMI >35 with medical problems. These problems include type 2 diabetes, high blood pressure, obstructive sleep apnea, nonalcoholic liver disease, osteoarthritis, high cholesterol, or heart disease. Patients who qualify for surgery often have tried various diets, exercise, and programs with some short-term weight loss but no long-term success. They may reach a plateau and get frustrated or not see enough response for the effort they feel they have put into weight loss. The mechanism of how bariatric surgery works is not completely understood. Some of the procedures work by restricting the amount of food consumed. Others cause restriction of calorie intake as well as changes in gut bacteria and hormones that alter appetite, satiety, and possibly metabolism (Apovian, Arrone, and Powell 2015; NHLBI 2012). Surgery, though successful in decreasing weight significantly, does have risk. It is important to understand the procedure and the potential risk and benefits. Additionally, after surgery the total amount of weight loss depends in large part on the changes a person makes and is able to maintain in regards to diet, exercise, and behavior modification. Before considering surgery as an option, you should think about the following questions and discuss them with your doctor:

1. Have you tried to lose weight and have been unsuccessful or unable to sustain the weight loss?
2. Do you understand the procedure and its possible outcomes, including risk and benefits?
3. Are you ready to lose weight and change your life/health for the better?
4. Do you understand how the surgery will affect you and lead to changes in diet and portion limitations?
5. Have you considered the lifelong commitment to changing eating habits and being physically active?
6. Do you understand the need for medical follow-up and the need for extra vitamins?

Once these questions have been answered and the consequences fully understood, then you can move forward with bariatric surgery. There are four procedures available in the United States. Roux-en-Y gastric bypass (RYGB) surgery has been the most commonly performed, but the vertical-sleeve gastrectomy (VSG) has become more popular in recent years. The adjustable gastric band (AGB) has been very popular until more recently, as the VSG is becoming a preferred procedure. Lastly the biliopancreatic diversion with or without duodenal switch

(BPD or BPD/DS) is the least commonly performed. These procedures are performed under general anesthesia while you are asleep. The majority of these surgeries are performed laparoscopically with the use of small incisions and with the insertion of a camera and small tools. This leads to quicker recovery times and shorter hospital stays than open procedures. Bariatric surgery results in a smaller stomach or pouch and therefore limits the amount of food the stomach can hold.

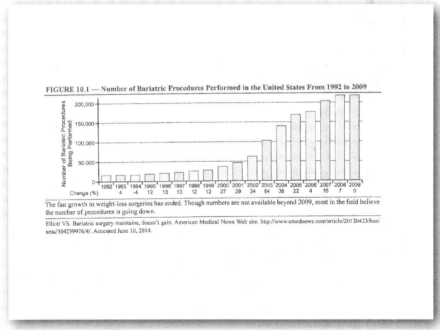

Figure 14. (Apovian, Arrone, and Powell 2015)

Roux-en-Y Gastric Bypass (RYGB)

The RYGB, or gastric bypass, is the most widely performed surgery and has been considered the standard of weight-loss surgeries. First the stomach is divided into two parts. The upper smaller pouch is where food enters the stomach, and it can only hold about one ounce of food. The pouch is about the size of a walnut. Secondly, the bypass involves taking a loop of the small intestine and attaching it to the pouch. Food eaten then travels from the stomach into the pouch and bypasses the first part of the gut, which absorbs a majority of nutrients from the food. The RYGB is considered a non-reversible procedure (NLM 2015). The RYGB results in loss of 60–80 percent of excess weight. With all procedures, there can be some weight regain of about 5 percent, but in the long term, it leads to >50 percent loss of extra body weight. It causes favorable changes in gut hormones that lead to satiety and also causes restriction in the amount of food that can be eaten. RYGB leads to greater remission of diabetes compared to other weight-loss surgeries. The cons of the surgery include long-term vitamin and mineral deficiencies with need for supplementation. Most common deficiencies are iron, vitamin D, vitamin B12, and zinc. RYGB requires lifelong vitamin/mineral supplementation as well as adherence to diet changes and follow-up with a physician (ASMBS 2016).

Vertical Sleeve Gastrectomy (VSG)

The VSG permanently removes about 80 percent of the stomach, leaving only a tube and is often referred to as the sleeve. The new pouch holds a much smaller amount of food than the normal stomach. This helps to decrease the number of calories/food that can be ingested. Similar to RYGB, this surgery alters the makeup of bacteria in the gut and the mix of gut hormones, leading to improvements in hunger, fullness, and control of blood sugar and cholesterol levels. VSG leads to rapid weight loss by restricting the amount of food passing through the stomach. It is similar to RYGB, with >50 percent of excess weight loss being maintained after three years. It does not require a change in how food passes through the intestines as with RGYB, and no foreign objects are inserted as with the AGB. Recovery is usually short with usually only a two-day hospital stay. Just like the RYGB, it is considered an irreversible procedure and can lead to vitamin deficiencies requiring supplements (ASMBS 2016).

Adjustable Gastric Band (AGB)

The AGB is often called the band, g-band, or lap band. It is performed laparoscopically and involves the placement of an inflatable band around the upper part of the stomach, creating a small pouch above the band. The anatomy of the stomach or the intestines is not altered as with the RYGB or VSG. The band works because the creation of the small pouch means only a small amount of food causes fullness very quickly. The size of the stomach opening can be adjusted over time through a port that sits under the skin in the abdominal area. The port is injected with a saline solution that is used to inflate the band. The band size is adjusted over time until there is a point reached that allows food restriction without vomiting of food.

The band is restrictive. This means it restricts the amount of food that can pass through into the stomach and gut at one time. It does not cause malabsorption of nutrients but seems to decrease hunger. The AGB leads to weight loss of about 40–50 percent, which is less than the weight loss seen with either the RYGB or VSG. However, it has less risk of complications after surgery or vitamin deficiencies compared to the other procedures. The hospital stay is very short—usually less than one day. The band procedure can be reversed if needed and is adjustable, as mentioned.

Problems with the procedure are that one sees less early weight loss, and the weight loss is slower. Less people lose at least 50 percent of excess body weight compared to other procedures, and it has the highest rate of reoperation. Potential side effects include erosion of the band into the stomach or slipping of the band. Rarely mechanical problems with the band or the port can occur (Apovian, Arrone, and Powell 2015; WIN, n.d.).

Biliopancreatic Diversion with or without Duodenal Switch (BPD, BPD/DS)

BPD/DS is a two-step procedure that is not commonly performed in the United States. It is a two-step procedure that involves first the creation of a small tubular stomach pouch similar to the VSG. Then about three-fourths of the small intestine is bypassed, and the lower part of the small intestine is brought up and connected to the stomach pouch. BPD differs from RYGB or other procedures because a large portion of the intestine is bypassed, and food does not mix with digestive enzymes until far down in the small intestine. This anatomic change leads to significant decrease in the absorption of calories and nutrients (Noria and Grantcharov 2013).

BPD/DS leads to changes in gut hormones along with decreased appetite and satiety similar to the other procedures. It leads to greater weight loss than RYGB, VSG, or AGB, with patients having a loss of 60–70 percent excess weight or more at a five-year follow-up. It is the most effective in leading to remission of diabetes and allows patients to eventually eat near "normal" meals (Apovian, Arrone, and Powell 2015). One must consider, however, the higher complication rate and risk of mortality compared to other surgeries. There is a longer hospital stay and great potential for not only vitamin and mineral deficiencies but also protein deficiency. This surgery requires strict follow-up as well as adherence to diet and vitamin supplementation.

The overall mortality (death rate) for bariatric surgery is <1 percent. However, side effects or adverse reactions can occur in as many as 20 percent of cases. Despite the risk, bariatric surgery is more effective for weight loss than diet, exercise, and medications combined, which can result in 5–11 percent weight loss commonly and (rarely) up to 14–20 percent weight loss. It is the only treatment available that can lead to long-term diabetes remission without medication. Bariatric surgery leads to significant reductions in blood pressure, cholesterol, and it greatly decreases the risk associated with obesity.

Overall bariatric-surgery procedures are safe. When it comes to safety, the thirty-day mortality for bariatric surgery ranges from 0.1 to 2 percent (Apovian, Arrone, and Powell 2015; Poirier et al. 2011; Tice et al. 2008). AGB has the lowest mortality rate (0.1 percent), whereas RYGB and VSG have a mortality rate of about 0.5 percent. The mortality rate depends on a number of factors, including the type of operation, patient's medical problems, and the surgeon's experience.

Mortality tends to be higher for those who are older, have complex medical problems, or are extremely obese, with BMI ≥50.

As mentioned briefly in the beginning, obesity is also an epidemic among children and teenagers. Although it has started to decline, some in the past few years, it still affects a large proportion of the population. According to the CDC website, 12.7 million children aged two to nineteen years are obese. That is approximately 17 percent of children who are obese and at risk for early development of diabetes and its consequences (CDC 2015). Just as it is hard for adults to lose weight, it can be hard for children as well. Bariatric surgery has been evaluated and is a possible treatment for select obese adolescents. Currently studies are underway, and short-term data shows early safety in this population after surgery. Studies are still ongoing in order to give us answers about long-term safety and effectiveness.

So what happens after surgery? People who undergo bariatric surgery need to be followed by a physician long term. After surgery, people are monitored for complications and weight loss in the first year. As mentioned before, vitamin deficiencies and nutritional issues may develop in the first year. Complications in the beginning can include nausea/vomiting, wound infections, or blockages of the intestines or stomach, depending on the type of surgery.

Later on patients have to focus on weight maintenance because they can regain some of the weight originally lost, especially if they do not adhere to dietary changes and an exercise regimen. People have to continue vitamin and mineral supplementation as prescribed, or significant deficiencies can occur. Other long-term complications include development of gallstones, dumping syndrome in RYGB, and persistent vomiting. Women should avoid pregnancy within eighteen months of surgery due to rapid weight loss and nutrition requirements. All patients should stop smoking and drinking alcohol because of negative consequences of both.

In short, bariatric surgery has flourished and continued to improve since it was first introduced in the 1950s. There are a variety of procedures available, and the best weight-loss surgery for a person should depend on his or her risk, amount of weight loss needed, and a detailed conversation with a physician of the risks and benefits. Bariatric surgery, whether RYGB, VSG, AGB, or BPD/DS, is proven to result in significant weight loss and improvements in diabetes, sleep apnea, hypertension, and cholesterol. Exactly how these metabolic changes occur are still being researched and thought to be due to changes in hormones and favorable changes in gut bacteria. Bariatric surgery overall is a good and viable option for select people.

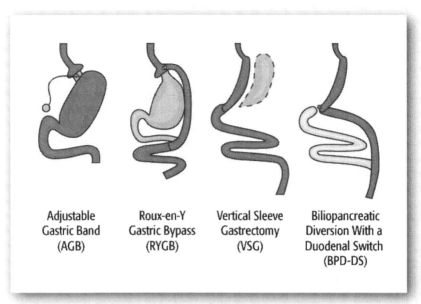

Figure 15. Options for bariatric surgery.

Image retrieved from

http://www.niddk.nih.gov/health-information/health-topics/weight-control/bariatric-surgery-severe-obesity/Pages/bariatric-surgery-for-severe-obesity.aspx.

Surgery is an excellent treatment for obesity but it is not for everyone. As the obesity epidemic becomes wider spread new treatments and procedures are being developed. Here is a brief discussion of newer treatments and procedures that are now available or being researched currently. The gastric balloon is a device inserted by a special medical device with a camera called an endoscope. The procedure is performed by a trained gastroenterologist and involves the inflation of a balloon into the stomach that is then inflated. The inflated balloon limits the amount of food that can enter and pass through the stomach. The device remains in place for up to six months and is later removed by endoscope. The gastric balloon originally introduced in 1985 but there were problems with the balloon deflating. Newer products have revamped the gastric balloon and try to address this problem. The FDA has approved a product call Obera, which is an alternative to bariatric surgery. It is a device comprised of two balloons that are inserted into the stomach and inflated by a trained gastroenterologist. If one balloon deflates ideally the other will remain inflated. Side effects most commonly include stomach pain, nausea, heart burn and less commonly more serious reactions such as ulcers, migration of the balloon and bowel obstruction. Various studies have showed an average weight loss range of 20-40 pounds depending on the duration of use of the balloon.

The Maestro Rechargeable System is another weight loss device approved by the FDA in 2015. This device is for use in obese adults with a BMI of thirty-five to forty-five. Think of it as a pacemaker that blocks the signals from the brain to the vagus nerve which regulates hunger and satiety. It is a surgically implanted device placed just under the skin. It sends electrical pulses to the vagus never and can be customized to as needed by a health care professional. The system is rechargeable and does not alter one's anatomy. It can be adjusted or removed as desired.

CHAPTER 13
Patients' Success Stories

As endocrinologists, we see people all the time who want to lose weight or have had trouble losing weight despite changes in diet and exercise. We see patients for various hormonal imbalances, and often patients just want to know why they cannot take off the extra pounds. We have helped several patients become successful in their weight-loss journey. Some were helped through addressing hormonal problems and others through advice on food intake, exercise, and the use of medications. For those reasons we started a weight-loss program in our office called Weigh Less for Way Less. Here are just a few examples of patients we have helped and those who inspire us to continue to work with people who struggle with weight.

JW was a forty-six-year-old man who presented to the clinic in January 2013 because he was frustrated with his lack of weight loss after years of trying various things. He was not able to do much physical activity due to lack of energy and weakness. He tried the low-carb diet, Atkins diet, and the South Beach diet in the past. The various diets worked for him initially with small amounts of weight loss, but as soon as he stopped the diet, he gained the weight back plus more. On presentation to the clinic, he weighed 350 pounds and was six feet three. His BMI was 39.7, which put him in the obese range.

He was examined and found to have signs of low testosterone. He was noted to have enlargement of the breast, and when asked about it, he reported noticing an increase in breast size. On further questioning, he reported some difficulty with sexual function. He was hesitant to discuss this at first but with some probing admitted to problems with libido and erections. When meeting with female doctors, men often are hesitant to admit when they have problems in the bedroom. However, JW was put at ease when he was jokingly told that doctors are like priests during confession. You can bare your soul without judgment, and it won't leave the room. That helped to ease the tension and establish the doctor-patient relationship and trust needed to help JW. Based on his complaints, symptoms, and physical exam, labs were ordered to determine hormone levels, including testosterone and other hormones, in order to figure out the underlying cause of his symptoms and inability to lose weight.

When endocrinologists evaluate hormone levels, we want to know if the problem is primary (from the gland itself) or secondary (from the pituitary gland—a small gland at the base of the brain) or if it is due to some other cause. The pituitary gland is considered the master gland. It is the control center for major organs such as the thyroid, adrenal gland, ovaries, and testes as well as a regulator for production and secretion of other hormones. Various illnesses can affect its function. After examining and talking to JW, labs were ordered to evaluate his pituitary function. Liver enzymes to rule out chronic disease of the liver and thyroid hormone levels were also examined because hypothyroidism can be a cause of low testosterone in some cases. The results came back about two weeks after his first visit. JW was anxious for the results, which revealed a very low testosterone level secondary to pituitary dysfunction. Further testing was done, and it revealed that JW had a pituitary tumor, which led to many of his symptoms. He was started on testosterone treatment. His tumor (a prolactinoma) did not need surgery and was treated with medication.

One month later, JW returned to the clinic and now weighed 315 pounds. He lost thirty-five pounds in two months. He reported feeling much better. He had improved energy and improvement in his libido and erectile dysfunction. With the positive changes, he gained confidence and started to exercise again. He started to build up muscle mass with his exercise. He was referred to the dietician and instructed on how to change his diet and portion sizes in ways that he could easily follow and keep up with long term. In 2014, he returned, and his weight was down to 289 pounds, and his BMI was 36.1. In 2015, he weighed 255 pounds with a BMI of 31.9 and had lost almost a hundred pounds since his initial visit. On his most recent visit, he was continuing to do well and has been able to continue to lose weight with treatment and changes in his diet and regular exercise. Most recently, he weighed in at 231 pounds and was feeling great. He continued to take testosterone replacement. He was happy that there was finally an answer to why he could not lose weight and that we were able to listen intently to his complaints and figure out that there was more to the picture. He had a happy ending to his long struggle and has changed not only his weight but also how he views his physical, emotional, and personal status. He was not told merely to have will power, which is what many people and even doctors might imply. Before saying *eat less and exercise more*, he was evaluated, and the root of the problem was discovered. When you get to the bottom of the problem, the weight loss will follow. JW continues to do well and is seen in clinic twice a year. He is aware that if anything changes, we will adjust his medications and provide support to help keep him on his weight-loss journey.

TS was a twenty-nine-year-old male when he came to the clinic for help. He had no significant medical problems but reported trouble with weight loss and was now concerned with enlargement of the breast (gynecomastia). He reported a past problem with gynecomastia during puberty, but it resolved on its own. More recently he noted enlargement of the breast again along with muscle weakness, fatigue (falling asleep at 8:00 p.m. every day), and his social life was nonexistent. He had become embarrassed to go out or even go to the gym because of his weight and physical appearance. He was five-feet-eleven with a weight of 234 pounds and BMI of 32.6.

At his first visit in July, a detailed history was taken, including his family history, detailed food journal, and his exercise regimen. Labs were also ordered to study his condition. His family history was positive for diabetes, high blood pressure, and high cholesterol. He was found to meet the criteria for metabolic syndrome. This is a syndrome that identifies people at risk for developing diabetes and its subsequent effects. He had a high waist circumference; his blood tests showed low HDL (good cholesterol), high triglycerides (types of fat); and he had abnormal liver function tests, which indicated fatty-liver disease or inflammation of the liver caused by excess deposit of fat in the liver. Given his lab results and family history, he was well on his way to developing full-blown diabetes in a few years.

Other labs showed that his testosterone was low, and the evaluation of the pituitary showed it to be working normally and that the problem was that his testes were not producing testosterone. He was started on medication for metabolic syndrome and testosterone. He was made aware of the risk and benefits of medication treatment and decided to go ahead with the recommended medications. At the start of treatment, his weight was 234 pounds. One month later his weight decreased to 208 pounds, and his BMI was 29.1. Three months later, he was down to 191 pounds with a BMI of 26.4. After four months, his weight was 183 pounds, BMI was 25.5, and at his most recent visit, he weighed 180 pounds with a BMI of 25.1. He was pleased with the results, and he now exercises regularly and has a girlfriend. His energy is improved. He can now stay awake at work, and he feels much better about himself. On repeat lab treatments, his cholesterol level normalized without cholesterol medicine, and his blood sugar was improved and is now in the normal range. He continues on treatment and is doing well. TS's case demonstrates that there can be other reasons contributing to obesity and its symptoms. We have to listen to the patient, and often the history and physical exam will give you a clue, if not an answer, to the patient's problem.

WJ was a fifty-four-year-old female first seen in October of 2014. She was referred by her primary-care doctor for uncontrolled diabetes and weight gain. She was 216 pounds with a height of five feet four and BMI of 37.1. She was diagnosed with type 2 diabetes two years before and was started on insulin for very high blood sugar. She was continued on insulin, and the dose was increased almost every two to three months. When she was first seen, she was on a total dose of 250 units of insulin. She was on two different types of insulin and taking four injections per day. She complained of feeling miserable and felt all she could focus on was her blood sugar and food. Taking so much insulin made her afraid to skip meals or try a low-carb diet due to concern for hypoglycemia (low blood sugar). Every time she took insulin, she noted an increase in her appetite. She was in a vicious cycle. She was getting more insulin to control the high blood sugar, which made her hungrier and led to weight gain, and the weight gain in turn led to more insulin resistance and the need for more insulin in order to try to overcome the resistance. She worked as a legal secretary and was sedentary sitting at a desk most of the day. Because of her fear of low BS or of making a mistake, she would keep food at her desk at work and constantly eat to try to avoid a low–blood sugar reaction while at work. When she was initially seen, she was noted to have a short neck with central obesity (most of the fat is concentrated in the middle), and she reported being depressed about going into retirement with nothing to look forward to other than checking her blood sugar and taking shots multiple times a day. Lab tests were done, and she was seen by a diabetes educator and dietician. The blood tests revealed that her pancreas was still working to produce insulin, and with many new diabetic medicines available, it was thought that she may not need insulin at such large doses. Her insulin was decreased to a long-acting insulin once a day, and the three injections with meals were stopped. She was given three newer medicines for blood sugar control.

Fortunately nowadays there are newer medicines for diabetes that are either weight neutral or can cause weight loss. Certain medicines take advantage of a hormone mentioned earlier called GLP-1 that is produced in the gut but acts on the brain to decrease the appetite as well as on the pancreas to help to control blood sugar. Another class of medicine works on the kidneys and causes the patient to get rid of sugar in the urine. It is like dumping sugar in the urine, and when you lose sugar, you lose calories. It leads to a loss of about three hundred to four hundred calories per day. Metformin is an old medicine that has been around for years and is part of first-line treatment in diabetes and helps to combat insulin resistance. WJ was excited to stop doing so many injections with the hope of not having to worry about her sugar dropping all the time. She was given a combination of the medicines along with a significant decrease in her insulin dosage, and in three weeks, she returned with weight down to 202 and BMI of 34.7. Three months later, she was able to stop insulin completely, and her weight was down to 178, and her BMI was 30.5. Another three months passed, and she continued to lose weight and was feeling much better. She was happier, feeling good about her body, and was exercising. She reported that her approach to food changed significantly, and she had an interesting way of measuring her appetite. She started to cut her meal in two parts. She would always eat the first part, and for the next six months, she would leave the rest for another meal. On her most recent visit, her weight was 145 pounds; and BMI, 24.9, which was in the normal range. Her hemoglobin A1C (a test that indicates one's average blood sugar) over three months was 6 percent. The goal for diabetics is usually less than 7 percent.

The next patient, KT, was a sixty-four-year-old female with a past history of thyroid disease. She was diagnosed with hypothyroidism (an underactive thyroid) after the birth of her last child almost twenty years earlier. She had been taking thyroid medication for many years and reported trouble with weight loss. She had been on the same dose of medicine for the past ten years. She was frustrated because she exercised, ate healthy, and was counting calories but found it hard to lose an extra ten to fifteen pounds that she gained over the years. On physical exam, she was noted to be short, and even a small amount of weight added extra pressure to her knees, making it more difficult for her to keep up a healthy lifestyle. This was frustrating to no end. Besides her history of thyroid disease and taking the medication, she had no other significant medical problems. KT was seen and examined, and she discussed her thyroid disease. It was explained to her that there is a wide range of normal for the thyroid-stimulating hormone (TSH), which is the test that is monitored for those with thyroid disease, and in most cases accurately reflects thyroid-hormone status. The range is 0.4–5, and many people function well in the midnormal range of 1–2, but some people feel better a little lower or higher. The bottom line is that different patients require different amounts of thyroid hormone, and having a normal level may not be normal for everyone. There is bell-shaped normal distribution. The majority of people fall in the middle range, but a small amount of people fall toward either end of the normal.

KT's TSH was 2.5–3 most of her life. Her dose was adjusted, and she was given a slightly higher dose. Her TSH was kept in the normal range, however. She felt better, and her weight started to decrease more easily. Her vitamin-D level was also normal, and she had improved energy and was able to achieve her weight-loss goal in about three months. She reported that she used to have mental fog, which is a common complaint in people with hypothyroidism and vitamin-D deficiency. She was another success in our clinic, and it only took listening and a few small changes to help her with her symptoms and to achieve her goal.

CHAPTER 14

Meal Plans

There is an enormous amount of information about what foods and diets are good for weight loss. These diets range from fad diets which are not recommended, to heavily researched diets such as low carb diets, low fat diets, high protein, vegetarian and diets high in fruits and vegetables with some lean protein. When you compare diets, low carb/high protein diets lead to quicker weight loss initially but over a longer period of six months all the diets end with similar amounts of weight loss. The key to long-term weight loss is not dieting and jumping onto the next hot trend but to change your habits for the long-run. This is what we call lifestyle changes. No diet is one-size fits all and no one diet works for everyone. Although one's weight is determined by a number of factors the basics of weight loss is to either eat less calories than you use or burn off more calories through exercise and activities than you intake. The recommended rate of weight loss is one to two pounds a week. That equates to a calorie deficit of 500 calories per day. At this rate weight loss can continue over a longer period of time. Faster weight loss is possible but it is harder to maintain larger calorie deficits over longer time periods. Before starting a reduced calorie diet consult your doctor to help determine you calorie needs and discuss with a registered dietician what type of diet is best for you. Included here are some examples of healthy diets for your information.

1200 Calorie Meal Plan

Meals	Example 1	Example 2
Breakfast		
	1 Starch: ½ cup of oatmeal or whole grain cereal	2 Starch: 2 slices of whole wheat toast
	1 Dairy: 8 oz cup of milk skim or 1%	1 Protein/fat: 2 tbsp peanut Butter
	1 Fruit: ½ banana or ¾ cup of berries	2 Fruit: 1 banana cut

Snack		
	1 fat: 10-12 almonds	1 Fruit: ½ grapefruit
Lunch		
	1 Starch: 1 slice whole grain bread	1 Starch: 1 slice whole grain bread
	2 Meat, lean: 2oz smoked salmon	2 Meat, lean: 2oz sliced turkey breast
	1 Fat: 1 tsp mayonnaise	1 Fat: 1tsp mayonnaise
	1 Vegetable: 1 cup tomato, cucumber, red onion salad	1 Vegetable: 1cup raw carrots
Snack		
	1 Fruit: small apple or orange	1 Dairy: 1 cup low-fat greek yogurt

Dinner		
	2 Starch: ½ cup of brown rice	2 starch: ½ baked sweet potato
	2 Meat: 2 oz baked chicken	2 Meat: 2oz grilled salmon
	2 vegetable: 1 cup sautéed spinach	2 vegetable: 1 cup cooked asparagus
	2 Fat: 2 tsp of olive oil	2 Fat: 2 tsp margarine for sweet potato

1500 Calorie Meal Plan

Meals	Example 1	Example 2
Breakfast		
	2 Starch: ½ cup of oatmeal 1 slice whole grain bread	1 Starch: 1 slices of whole wheat toast
	1 Fat: 6-8 almonds	1 Fat: 1 tsp butter
	1 Dairy: 1 cup greek yogurt	1 Protein/fat: 1 egg
	1 Fruit: ¾ cup of berries	1 Dairy: 1 cup milk skim or 1%
		2 Fruit: 1 banana cut
Snack		
	1 Fruit: 1 small pear	1 Vegetable: 1 cup celery with 1 tsp peanut butter

Lunch		
	2 Starch: 2 slices whole grain bread	2 Starch: 2 slices whole grain bread
	2 Meat, lean: 2oz chicken	2 Meat, lean: 2oz sliced turkey breast
	1 Fat: 1 tsp mayonnaise	1 Fat: 1tsp mayonnaise
	1 Vegetable: ½ cup sliced tomato and 2 leaves of lettuce	1 fruit: 1cup strawberries
Snack		
	1 Fruit: 1 & ¼ cups watermelon	1 Dairy: 1 cup low-fat greek yogurt

Dinner		
	2 Starch: ½ cup of Corn, 1 small dinner roll	2 starch: ½ large baked potato
	3 Meat: 3 oz baked chicken	3 Meat: 3oz steak, broiled or grilled
	2 vegetable: 1 cup cooked broccoli	2 vegetable: 1 cup cooked Green beans
	2 Fat: 2 tsp of olive oil	2 Fat: 1 tbsp butter for potato

1800 Calorie Meal Plan

Meals	Example 1	Example 2
Breakfast		
	1 Starch: 1 slice of whole grain toast	2 Starch: ½ cup of oatmeal 1 slice whole wheat toast
	2 Protein: 1 egg, 1 chicken sausage link	1 Fat: 1 tbsp chopped walnuts
	1 Dairy: 8 oz cup of greek yogurt	1 Fruit: ¾ cup of blueberries
	1 tsp margarine or butter	1 Dairy: 8 oz cup of skim milk
	1 Fruit: ½ cup of raspberries	

Snack		
	1 Fruit: 1 cup cubed cantaloupe	1 Protein: ¼ cup low-fat cottage cheese
Lunch		
	2 Starch: 2 slices whole grain bread	1 Starch: 1 slice whole grain bread
	3 Meat, lean: ¾ cup tuna (canned in water)	3 Meat, lean: 3 oz sliced turkey breast
	2 Fat: 1 tsp mayonnaise 1 tbsp Italian dressing	1 Fat: 1tsp mayonnaise
	1 Vegetable: 1 cup mixed greens salad	1 Vegetable: 1cup raw Carrots
		1 Fruit: ¾ cup fresh pineapple

Snack		
	1 Fruit: 1 Kiwi	1 Fat: 1 tbsp peanut butter
	1 Protein: ¼ cup of low-fat cottage cheese	1 fruit: 1 small apple cut into slices

Dinner		
	2 Starch: 1 cornbread 2 inch Square	2 starch: ⅔ cup of cooked lentils, ¾ cup butternut squash
	3 Meat: 3 oz lean pork chop grilled or baked	3 Meat: 3oz broiled tilapia
	2 vegetable: 1 cup cooked cabbage	2 vegetable: 1 cup cooked broccoli
	2 Fat: 1tbsp of margarine	2 Fat: 2 tsp olive oil
	1 Fruit: 1 cup cantaloupe/honey dew melon	1 Fruit: 1 Peach

Snack		
	1 Starch: 3 cups popcorn	1 Starch: 7 dried apricot halves
	1 Protein: 1 oz lean roast beef	1 Fat: 1 handful mixed nuts
	1 Dairy: 1 slice cheese	1 Dairy: 1 packet hot cocoa

2000 Calorie Meal Plan

Meals	Example 1	Example 2
Breakfast		
	2 Starch: ½ cup of grits, 1 slice whole grain toast	2 Starch: 2 frozen whole grain waffles
	1 Fat: 1 tsp margarine	2 Protein/fat: 2 tbsp peanut Butter
	2 Fruit: 1 small orange, ½ Cup apple juice	1 Fruit: ½ banana
		1 Dairy: 8 oz cup of milk Skim or 1%
Snack		
	1 Protein: 1 oz lunch meat	1 Protein: 1 boiled egg
	1 Dairy: 1 oz slice of cheese	

Lunch		
	3 Starch/Protein: 2 cups chicken noodle soup, 6 saltine crackers	3 Starch: 1 pita bread, 2tbsp
		2 Meat, lean: 2oz chicken strips
	2 Vegetable: small garden salad	
		1 Fat: 1tbsp lemon vinaigrette
	2 Fat: 2 tbsp. Balsamic vinaigrette	1 Vegetable: 1 cup Greek salad
Snack		
	1 Fruit: 12 medium grapes	1 Fruit: 2 small tangerines

Dinner		
	2 Starch: 1 cornbread 2inch square 1 corn on the cob-6 inch Piece	3 starch: 2 tortillas, 1/3 cup cooked rice
	3 Meat: 3 oz. broiled lamb chops	2 Meat: 2oz grilled shrimp
	3 vegetable: 1 cup cooked collard greens, ½ cup sautéed mushrooms	3 vegetable: 1 cup grilled onions and peppers, ⅓ cup chopped tomato, ½ cup shredded lettuce
	2 Fat: 2 tsp of salad dressing and mixed green salad	2 Fat/Dairy: 1 oz. shredded Cheese, 1 tbsp. guacamole

Snack		
	1 Fruit: 12 cherries	2 Starch: ½ cup of fruit Sorbet
	1 Starch: 3 graham cracker Squares	1 Fat: 1 tbsp. chopped nuts
	1 Protein/fat: 1 tbsp. almond or peanut butter	

CHAPTER 15

The Elephant in the Room: Why We Wrote This Book

How many times have you gone to the doctor's office, and the doctor never discussed your weight? So many diseases are treated every day, and millions of dollars are spent on obesity-related health issues, yet very few physicians are addressing the underlying problem. As endocrinologists, we see all the effort put into treating diabetes and developing new medicines for control. However, until recent years, there has been a real shortage in medications to treat and address underlying problems leading to obesity. Many professional medical societies and associations talk about treating diabetes but not about the underlying cause: obesity!

Numerous doctors treat and replace joints affected by arthritis caused by excess weight daily, but still the cause goes unaddressed. If weight is mentioned as the cause, the advice is simply to lose weight, without any guidance. The same goes for heart disease, which is the number-one killer of Americans, and also for stroke. We can go on and on about all the different diseases that are caused by obesity, but the last thing to be addressed is weight loss. Screening is easy to do because patients are always weighed when they go to the doctor. With the exception of the ophthalmologists' and dermatologists' offices, it is standard practice for patients to be weighed and the BMI to be calculated. We already have the information at hand, and we physicians have to make a more conscious effort to address the elephant in the room that everybody sees but nobody wants to talk about. It is important because diabetes, cancer, and obesity are things that can be avoided. These words take on action and can impact and affect our lives significantly. Americans are living longer, but we want you to live better. The best way to do that is to be healthy.

An increasing number of medical societies are recognizing obesity as a disease that should be addressed and treated. Articles are being published, and news headlines in journals, the Internet, and television are reporting regularly about obesity and its effects.

Here are some headlines published in *Endocrine News* just this year:

Despite Massive Efforts, Obesity on the Rise in the US June 2016

See more at http://endocrinenews.endocrine.org/despite-massive-efforts-obesity-on-the-rise-in-the-u-s/#sthash.ew9rfo6h.dpuf.

Tendency to Obesity and Diabetes Can Be Inherited May 2016
See more at http://endocrinenews.endocrine.org/tendency-to-obesity-and-diabetes-can-be-inherited/#sthash.UK2eo4wA.dpuf.

The Epigenetics of Obesity
By Eric Seaborg, February 2016
"Obesity appears to change genetic expression in ways that favor the development of diabetes and other conditions—changes that might even be passed on to the next generation." See more at http://endocrine-news.endocrine.org/the-epigenetics-of-obesity/#sthash.F80W2Jag.dpuf.

Obesity has become an epidemic and because of that, a new society was created: the Obesity Society. It is a scientific society that seeks to advance the understanding of the causes, consequences, treatment, and prevention of obesity.

Efforts to bring awareness of obesity, the disease, led to the establishment of the Obesity Action Coalition (OAC). The OAC is a nonprofit organization dedicated to helping people understand the causes and treatments related to obesity and offering support for people along the way. They seek to make the conversation larger and louder in order to decrease bias and discrimination for people and, in short, to help people deal with the significant impact obesity has on health.

We feel the same. We see so many people just getting by with aches, pains, and fatigue who are not enjoying life to the fullest. They neither see a way out of their predicament nor know how to change lifelong habits of eating, overindulging, and not being active that have been ingrained often since childhood. The good news is that there is help available, and weight loss is not impossible. Physicians should first do no harm, but if doing nothing is also harmful, that is not acceptable. We wanted to take action to inform people of the problems associated with obesity and the reasons people often fail. We hoped to highlight how the endocrine system plays into all this and, above all, to set people on the path to better health.

REFERENCES

American Society for Metabolic and Bariatric Surgery. n.d. "Bariatric Surgery Procedures." https://asmbs.org/patients/bariatric-surgery-.

Apovian, Caroline M., Louis Arrone, and Amanda G. Powell. 2015. *Clinical Management of Obesity*. West Islip, NY: Professional Communications Inc.

Beccuti, Gugliemo, and Silvana Pannain. 2011. "Sleep and Obesity." *Current Opinion in Clinical Nutrition and Metabolic Care* 14 (4): 402–12.

CDC. Updated June 19, 2015. "Childhood Obesity Facts." http://www.cdc.gov/obesity/data/childhood.html.

Donnelly, Joseph E., Steven N. Blair, John M. Jakicic, Malinda M. Manore, Janet W. Rankin, and Byran K. Smith. 2009. "Appropriate Physical Activity Intervention Strategies for Weight Loss and Prevention of Weight Regain for Adults." American College of Sports Medicine. *Medicine & Science in Sports & Exercise* 41:459–71.

Flegal, Katherine M., Margaret D. Carroll, Cynthia L. Ogden, and Clifford L. Johnson 2002. "Prevalence and Trends in Obesity among US Adults, 1999–2000." *JAMA* 288:1723–7.

Ford, Earl S., David F. Williamson, and Simin Liu. 1997. "Weight Change and Diabetes Incidence: Findings from a National Cohort." *American Journal of Epidemiology* 146:214–22.

Garber, Carol Ewing, Bryan Blissmer, Michael R. Deschenes, Barry A. Franklin, Michael J. Lamonte, I-Min Lee, David C. Nieman, and David P. Swain. 2011. "Quantity and Quality of Exercise for Developing and Maintaining Cardiorespiratory, Musculoskeletal, and Neuromotor Fitness in Apparently Healthy Adults: Guidance for Prescribing Exercise." American College of Sports Medicine. *Medicine & Science in Sports & Exercise* 43:1334–9.

Girardin, Jean- Louis, Natasha J. Williams, Daniel Sarpong, Abhishek Pandey, Shawn Youngstedt, Ferdinand Zizi, and Gbenga Ogedegbe. 2014. "Associations between Inadequate Sleep and Obesity in the US Adult Population: Analysis of the National Health Interview Survey (1977–2009)." *BMC Public Health* 14:290.

Higgins, John P., and Christopher L. Higgins. 2016. "Prescribing Exercise to Help Your Patients Lose Weight." *Cleveland Clinic Journal of Medicine* 83 (2): 141–50.

Kahan, Scott. 2015. "The Landscape of Obesity Pharmacotherapy: Surveying the Options." *Obesity Consultants* 3 (1): 9–13.

Khaodhiar, Lalita, Sue Cummings, and Caroline M. Apovian. 2009. "Treating Diabetes and Prediabetes by Focusing on Obesity Management." *Current Diabetes Reports* 9 (5): 348–54.

Medline Plus website. 2015. "Gastric Bypass Surgery." https://www.nlm.nih.gov/medlineplus/ency/article/007199.htm.

NHLBI Obesity Education Initiative. 2012. "The Practical Guide: Identification, Evaluation, and Treatment of Overweight and Obesity in Adults." http://www.nhlbi.nih.gov/files/docs/guide-lines/prctgd_c.pdf.

Noria, Sabrina F., and Teodor Grantcharov. 2013 "Biological Effects of Bariatric Surgery on Obesity-related Comorbidities." *Canadian Journal of Surgery* 56 (1): 47–57.

Obesity: Preventing and Managing the Global Epidemic. 2000. Report of a WHO Consultation. *World Health Organ Technical Report Series* 894. i–xii:1–253.

Ogden, Cynthia L., Margaret D. Carroll, and Brian K. Kit, Katherine M. Flegal. 2014. "Prevalence of Childhood and Adult Obesity in the United States, 2011–2012." *JAMA* 311 (8): 806–14.

Poirier, Paul, Marc-Andre Cornier, Theodore Mazzone, Sasha Stiles, Susan Cummings, Samuel Klein, Peter A. McCullough, Christine Ren Felding, and Barry A. Franklin. 2011. "Bariatric Surgery and Cardiovascular Risk Factors: A Scientific Statement from the American Heart Association." *Circulation* 123 (15): 1683–701.

Reddon, Hudson, Hertzel C. Gerstein, James C. Engert, Viswanathan Mohan, Jackie Bosch, Dipika Desai, Swneke D. Bailey, Rafael Diaz, Salim Yusuf, Sonia S. Anand, and David Meyre. 2016. "Physical Activity and Genetic Predisposition to Obesity in a Multiethnic Longitudinal Study." *Scientific Reports* 6:18672.

Rosenberg, Michael M. 1998. "Weight Change with Oral Contraceptive Use and during the Menstrual Cycle: Results of Daily Measurements." *Contraception* 58 (6): 345–49.

Ryan, Donna H., and Holly R. Wyatt. 2015. "Assessing the Underlying Pathophysiological Processes Associated with Obesity." *Obesity Consults* 3 (1): 4–8.

Schwartz, Alexander, and Eric Doucet. 2010. "Relative Changes in Resting Energy Expenditure During Weight Loss: A Systematic Review." *Obesity Review* 11:531–47.

Stoeckel, Luke E., Rosalyn E. Weller, Edwin W. Cook III, Donald B. Twiegb, Robert C. Knowltonc, and James E. Cox. 2008. "Widespread Reward-System Activation in Obese Women in Response to Pictures of High-Calorie Foods." *Neuroimage* 41 (2): 636–47.

The Weight-Control Information Network (WIN) website. n.d. "Bariatric Surgery for Severe Obesity." https://www.niddk.nih.gov/health-information/health-topics/weight-corol/bariatric-surgery/Pages/overview.aspx.

Tice, Jeffery A., Leah Karliner and Judith Walsh, Amy J. Petersen, and Mitchell D. Feldman. 2008. "Gastric Banding or Bypass? A Systematic Review Comparing the Two Most Popular Bariatric Procedures." *American Journal of Medicine* 121:885–93.

Timpson, Nicholas J., Pauline M. Emmett, Timothy M. Frayling, Imogen Rogers, Andrew T. Hattersley, Mark I. McCarthy, and George Davey Smith. 2008. "The Fat Mass- and Obesity-Associated Locus and Dietary Intake in Children." *American Journal of Clinical Nutrition* 88 (4): 253–62.

Vrbikova, Jana, Katerina Dvorakova, Martin Hill, and Luboslav Starka. 2006. "Weight Change and Androgen Levels during Contraceptive Treatment of Women Affected by Polycystic Ovary." *Endocrine Regulations* 40:119–23.

Wadden, Thomas A., Robert I. Berkowitz, Leslie G. Womble, David B. Sarwer, Suzanne Phelan, Robert K. Cato, Louise A. Hesson, Suzette Y. Osei, Rosalind Kaplan, and Albert J. Stunkard. 2005. "Randomized Trial of Lifestyle Modification and Pharmacotherapy for Obesity." *New England Journal of Medicine* 35:2111–20.

ACKNOWLEDGMENTS

I would like to thank all the people who helped me with the idea, development, and production of this book. First I thank Dr. Washington for writing this book with me. Thanks go to my office manager, Lety, for taking care of all the important details and allowing me time to think bigger. I thank Irma, our Weigh Less for Way Less program director, for her help. I thank all my patients for trusting me with their care and pushing me to publish this book.

MAHA ABBOUD

I would like to thank all the people who encouraged me and were excited for me from the start of this book idea. I feel very passionate about eating healthy, exercise, and weight loss because I have seen all the bad outcomes that can occur when this important issue of obesity is overlooked. I want to thank my father for always giving me advice and preaching to the choir. He has struggled with obesity and diabetes for a large part of his adult life. I appreciate his excitement for me and his encouragement throughout the process of writing this book. I thank my mother for correcting my grammar. As a retired high-school English teacher, she was instrumental in proofreading and keeping me on point. I want to thank my sister for her invaluable opinions. I thank you, my family, for your love and encouragement.

TERRI WASHINGTON